Herbal Healing Inheritance

The layman's key to identify common complaints and how to treat them with herbs.

BRITISH MEDICAL JOURNAL, 26th FEBRUARY, 1916

Excellent Herbs had our fathers of old
Excellent Herbs to ease their pain –
Alexanders and Marigolds,
Eyebright, Orris and Elecampane,
Basil, Rocket, Valerian, Rue
(Almost singing themselves they run)
Vervain, Dittany, 'Call-me-to-you'
Cowslip, Melilot, Rose-of-the-sun;
Anything green that grew out of the mould;
Was an excellent Herb to our fathers of old.

Rudyard Kipling.

Herbal Healing Inheritance

by

Dr. Bessie Howarth, M.B., C.H.B., M.N.I.M.H.

*Physician and Surgeon, Consultant Herbal Practitioner,
Member of the National Institute of Medical Herbalists*

Regency Press (London & New York) Ltd.
125 High Holborn, London WC1V 6QA

**DEDICATED TO
CHARLES AND DOMENIC
ALWAYS 'PILLARS OF STRENGTH'**

ISBN 0 7212 0860 6

Printed and bound in Great Britain by
Buckland Press Ltd., Dover, Kent.

Contents

Foreword

On compiling this publication my mother felt that she was able to provide a bridge to link her two lifelong interests, namely herbs and their medicinal qualities and orthodox medicine which she has practised for over forty years.

Her formative years, back in the days leading up to and through the First World War were spent with the lingering scent of new-mown hay and the hanging perfumes of May Blossom and Wild Honeysuckle and the scents of the many wild flowers that adorned the fields on those warm summer days. These are her vivid childhood memories.

We are of 'farming' stock with a family history dating back over the past 400 years. Our forbears farmed the Pennine Slopes and the Flat Lands of Lancashire.

She reflects fondly on the lunch-time 'breaks' at haymaking time with the herb beer and chunks of hard cheese and the chances she had as a child to sit, to muse, and become as one with her surroundings as Alice might have done in her Wonderland. She pictures the coloured flower-heads waving backwards and forwards and gently nodding to the delicate breezes on those summer days in the shimmering heat.

Her father, my grandfather, was a taskmaster of the best kind, dedicated to his daily work and the welfare of his family. His strict Victorian values dictated that his children all knew how to farm satisfactorily, whether boy or girl, as was the family tradition, and in addition, to carry on enthusiastically with school work and education.

His children, in their later years, voiced eternal thanks for his foresight and dedication. Her mother, my grandmother churned the milk and made the butter and cheese, and 'batches' of home-made bread – there were five surviving children to be catered for. My mother has said that my grandmother was the kind of woman who gave her the greatest gift that she possessed, and that was an appreciation of the little things in life.

It was amongst these rigid Victorian values and the charm of pear blossom time that a compromise was born in my mother. She recalls the pear tree growing up the walls of the house and the branches with blossom, actually invading her bedroom window.

Her love of all things that were around her was encouraged by her parents. She would spend many 'ecstatic' hours, as a child riding up and down a cinder path along with her sisters and brother on a tyre-less boneshaker bicycle. They were not rich. Many people were poor in those days, but at the risk of a cliche, they were very happy. They did not count their riches as the money in their pockets or their material possessions, but in the ever-changing moods of nature, the calls as to whether the mornings were frosty and bracing, or warm and relaxing, the beauty of the setting sun, and the glory of a sunrise heralding a new day. Their riches were the visiting magpies chattering endlessly in the tall poplar trees, or the kingfisher diving for 'tiddlers' in the pond behind the house. Even to this day she still finds the haunting call of the rooks in the high tree-tops most relaxing.

Nature gives so much to the discerning eye and asks so little in return. It was from this background and with some enthusiasm that she decided a 'Vet's' life was for her. She was fortunate in that she had apparently shown enough mental capacity to make a university place a possibility, but what nature had credited her with, intellectually, she had unfortunately seemed fit to debit her physically, and at barely 5 ft. tall it seemed to my grandfather a 'tall' order or lack of one that she should find herself tackling a cow with a difficult birth, or getting to grips with an obstinate boar. The solution was going to be 'Medicine' where she could treat her fellow men with the same enthusiasm she was prepared to treat her fellow beasts.

Yet again, she was fortunate in that the university she had chosen, and had boasted such a fine veterinary school, also had an equally talented medical department, and Liverpool was within reach, though I would reflect carefully before I added the word 'easy' as she had to cycle, for a period of one whole year, a round trip of 44 miles per day from her home in Leigh, and then had to settle down to study each evening. Her education kept her fit! I wonder how many can boast that today.

After 40 years she still says that her alternative choice was a good one. After qualifying as a doctor in orthodox medicine in 1939 at the age of 26 years, she joined the Indian Medical Service at the outbreak of the Second World War and was stationed in the foothills of the Himalayas at a place called Naini Tal. She still recalls the thrill of the rising sun lighting up the snow-clad slopes of Kanchenjunga – the second highest peak in the Himalayan range, reminding her of the pink sugar mice given as a Christmas treat to the children. She has always been with Nature for it has always given her so much pleasure. She quotes Tennyson and repeats:–

'Little flower if I could understand what you are, root and all
I should know what God and man are.'

To become familiar with the 'medicinal' side of the herbs she so much appreciated, she attended the School of Herbal Medicine in Tunbridge Wells, Kent, and qualified as a Consultant Herbal Practitioner in 1978. She ran both an orthodox and a herbal practice for a few years in the North of England and retired to live in Devon where she found she had the urge to compile this book, to inspire future generations in the scientific research of further knowledge in the value of herbs for the benefit of mankind.

C. Zacchia.

Herb Farms and Suppliers

D   Herb Society members given 10% discount.
P   Postal service available.

Herb Farms

D   **Askett Nurseries,** Flowery Field, Askett, Nr. Aylesbury, Bucks. HP17 9LY. Tel. (08444) 6356. Herbs, heathers, perennials, etc. Retail and wholesale. Van delivery service.

P   **Binks Nurseries,** Darlington Road, Northallerton, North Yorkshire. Tel. (0609) 3992.

PD **Bowling Alley Herb Farm,** Commonside, Alvanley, Via Warrington, Cheshire. Tel. (09284) 285. Dried herbs and spices, farmhouse and own make herb cheese.

D   **Brin School Fields,** The Old School, Flichity, Inverness. Tel. (08083) 288.

D   **Brookside Herbs,** Brookside, Walgrave Road, Hannington, Northampton NN6 9SX. Tel. (0604) 781593. Herb garden, herbs and wild flowers. Please telephone before visiting.

PD **Candlesby Herbs,** Cross Keys Cottage, Candlesby, Spilsby, Lincs. Tel. Scremby (075485) 211. Aromatics and culinary products. Lectures and broadcasting.

PD **Caroline Holmes – Herbs,** Denham End Farm, Denham, Bury St. Edmunds, Suffolk IP29 5EE. Tel. (0284) 810653. Day courses, group visits, lectures and talks.

Cheshire Herbs, Fourfields, Forest Road, Little Budworth, Nr. Tarporley, Cheshire CW6 9ES. Tel. (082921) 578. Herb garden, shop selling herb related products, talks, group visits.

PD **Chiltern Country Herbs,** Trinity Farm House, 49 Worminghall Road, Oakley, Nr. Aylesbury, Bucks. Tel. (0844) 238020. A postal gift service – 'You Choose, We Send'.

PD **Cornish Herbs,** Trelow Cottage, Mawgan-in-Meneage, Nr. Helston, Cornwall. Tel. Mawgan 374. Herb nursery, gardens, shop. Catalogue for 3 x 2nd class stamps.

D **The Cottage Herbery,** Mill House, Boraston, Nr. Tenbury Wells, Worcs. Tel. (058479) 575. Herb garden, shop, day schools. 3 x 1st class stamps for catalogue.

PD **Deepdale Organic Growers.** Wheal Francs, Goonhavern, Nr. Truro, Cornwall TR4 9NR. Tel. (0872) 54370. Organically grown vegetables.

Elidyr Nursery, Coleg Elidyr, Rhandirmwyn, Llandovery, Dyfed SA20 0NL. Tel. (05506) 272, Ext. 26. Crops of organic herb plants for cosmetics or homeopathic medicine.

D **Elly Hill Herbs,** Elly Hill House, Barmpton, Darlington, Co. Durham DL1 3JF. Tel. (0325) 464682. Conducted tour of herb garden with refreshments – see brochure.

PD **Fold Garden,** 26 Fold Lane, Biddulph, Staffs. ST8 7SG. Tel. (0782) 513028. Visits by appointment only. Groups catered for – S.A.E. for leaflet.

D **Foliage Scented and Herb Plants,** Walton Poor Cottage, Ranmore, Dorking, Surrey. Tel. (04865) 2273/4731. Garden open to public by appointment. Teas.

PD **Haddlesey Herb and Heather Centre,** West Haddlesey, Nr. Selby, North Yorks. YO8 8QA. Tel. (075 782) 279. Gardens designed, courses and talks, herbs in terracotta pots to order.

Heches Herbs, Les Heches, St. Peters, Guernsey, Channel Islands. Tel. (0481) 63545. Lecture holidays including an 'Introduction to Growing and Using Herbs'.

D **The Herb Farm,** Peppard Road, Sonning Common, Reading RG4 9NJ. Tel. (0734) 724220. Display gardens, plants, herb products, pots, containers, old barn shop.

D **The Herb Garden,** Hall View Cottage, Hardstoft, Pilsley, Nr. Chesterfield, Derbyshire. Tel. Chesterfield (0246) 854268. Herb garden and nursery open to public. Pot-pourri oils.

PD **The Herb Trust,** Littlecot House, Harpford, Sidmouth, Devon EX10 0NH. Tel. (0395) 68565. Culinary, medicinal and aromatic plants. Catalogue £1.30 including p & p.

PD **The Herbary Prickwillow,** Mile End, Prickwillow, Ely, Cambs. CB7 4SJ. Tel. Prickwillow (0353 88) 456. Herb garden, 3½ acre farm, refreshments, growing and cooking courses.

D **Hill Farm Herbs,** Hill Farm House, Park Walk, Brigstock, Northamptonshire. Tel. (0536) 73694. Nursery, tea room and shop, display gardens, pots and baskets.

PD **Hollington Nurseries Ltd.,** Woolton Hill, Newbury, Berks. Tel. (0635) 253908. Discount available to personal callers only.

PD **Iden Croft Herbs,** Frittenden Road, Staplehurst, Kent TN12 0DN. Tel. (0580) 891432. Herb gardens, plants, refreshments, shop. Garden for blind/disabled. Open all year.

PD **Lathbury Park Herbs,** Lathbury Park, Newport Pagnell, Bucks. Tel. (0908) 610316. Jams, pickles, pot-pourri, spices sold in addition to herbs.

D **Laurel Farm Herbs,** Main Road, Kelsale, Saxmundham, Suffolk IP17 2RG. Tel. Yoxford (072877) 223.

D **Lower Severalls Herb Nursery,** Lower Severalls, Crewkerne, Somerset. Tel. (0460) 73234. Herb garden illustrating ways of using herbs in garden design.

PD **Marle Place Plants,** Marle Place, Brenchley, Kent TN12 7HS. Tel. (089272) 2304. Wholesale retail herb plants, herb rockery. Garden open Wednesday p.m. Dried flowers, herbal goods, shop.

D **Mill Farm Pot-Pourri,** Wendling, Dereham, Norfolk NR19 2LY. Tel. Wendling (036 287) 211. Herb plants, pot-pourri, etc., Retail and wholesale. Herb garden.

D **Netherfield Herbs,** 37 Nether Street, Rougham, Bury St. Edmond, Suffolk. Tel. (0359) 70452. Herb garden open, lectures arranged, postal herb garden design service.

PD **Parkinson Herbs,** Barras Moor Farm, Perran ar Worthal, Truro, Cornwall. Tel. (0872) 864380. Lecture demonstrations throughout Cornwall. Herb products sold at nursery only.

D **Poplar Herb Farm,** Mark Road, Burtle, Nr. Bridgwater, Somerset. Tel. (0278) 723170. Herb plants and products. Astrological herb garden. S.A.E. for list.

PD **Salley Gardens,** 82 Julian Road, West Bridgford, Nottingham NG2 5AN. Tel. (0602) 810556. Rare medicinal and wildflower plants and seeds. S.A.E. for catalogue.

D **Samares Herbs à Plenty,** Samares Manor, St. Clement, Jersey, Channel Islands. Herb Shop, Herb Gardens, Herb Nursery. Tel. (0534) 79635. Herb talks and courses during tourist season April-October.

PD **Scotherbs,** Waterybutts, Grange by Errol, Perthshire PH2 7SZ. Tel. (082) 12228. Culinary herbs, S.A.E. for catalogue. Culinary herbs fresh cut and plants, herb based mustards, oils and vinegars.

PD **Sellet Hall Herb Garden,** Whittington, Nr. Kirkby Lonsdale, via Carnforth, Lancs. LA6 2QF. Tel. (0468) 71865. Display gardens of herbs and woodland plants, books and gifts.

PD **Selsley Herb & Goat Farm,** Waterlane, Selsley, Stroud, Gloucestershire. Tel. (04536) 6682. Herb gardens, animals to view and barn shop to browse in.

PD **Spots Farm Herb Garden,** Smallhythe, Tenterden, Kent TN30 7NG. Tel. (05806) 3033. Herb garden and vineyard open to public. Shop and bistro.

P **Suffolk Herbs.** Sawyers Farm, Little Cornard, Sudbury, Suffolk. Tel. (0787) 227247. Open Saturday only. Send S.A.E. for seeds by post catalogue.

PD **Waltham Herbs,** Waltham Windmill, Brigsley Road, Waltham, Lincs. Tel. Grimsby (0472) 814129. Landscape consultation, design and construction.

PD **Westhall Herbs,** Church Lane, Westhall, Nr. Halesworth, Suffolk IP19 8NU. Tel. Brampton (050279) 646. Herb teas, talks, garden design, books, pots, seeds, gifts.

PD **Yorkshire Herbs.** The Herb Centre, Middleton Tyas, Richmond, N. Yorks. DL10 6RR. Tel. (032577) 686. Wholesale/retail fresh cut herbs and herb plants.

Suppliers

P **Baldwins,** 173 Walworth Road, London, SE17. Tel. 01-703 5550. Tues. to Sats. 9.00 a.m. to 5.30 p.m. Closed Mondays. Mail order. S.A.E. for price list.

PD **Brome & Schimmer Ltd.,** Unit 3, Romsey Industrial Estate, Greatbridge Road, Romsey, Hants SO51 0HR. Tel. (0794) 515595. Culinary and medicinal herbs, spices, essential oils.

PD **Chanctonbury Herbs,** 104 High Street, Steyning, West Sussex BN4 3RD. Tel. (0903) 815000. Plants, herbal vinegars, mustards. Dried herbs and flowers. Own herbal cosmetics.

PD **Gaia Natural Therapies,** London Road, Forest Row, E. Sussex RH18 5EZ. Tel. (034282) 2716. S.A.E. for price list. Herbs, tinctures, essential oils, natural vitamins and supplements by post.

PD **Gerard House Ltd.,** 3 Wickham Road, Bournemouth BH7 6JX. Tel. (0202) 434116/7/8. Excellent range of herbal preparations and cosmetics, vitamins and minerals.

P **Hambleden Herbs,** Hambleden, Henley, Oxon RG9 6SX. Tel. (0491) 571598. Growers and importers of organic and wild-crafted dried herbs. Wholesale only.

D **Hartwood Aromatics,** Hartwood House, 12 Station Road, Hatton, Warwick CV35 7LG. Tel. (0926) 842873. Pure herbal essential oils, special remedy oils, body and skin oils. Aromatherapy books and supplies. Pot-pourri oils and porcelain oil burners.

PD **Little Herbs,** 1 West Street, Ware, Herts. SG12 9EE. Tel. (0920) 4054. Herbs, spices, fragrant gifts, herbal cosmetics, aromatherapy supplies, dried flowers.

PD **Phoenix International Health Books and Herbs,** Aston House, 26 Kingston Road, New Malden, Surrey KT3 3LS. Tel. (London) 01-942 5668. 24 hour service as far as possible.

P **Potters (Herbal Supplies) Ltd.,** Leyland Mill Lane, Wigan. Tel. (0942) 34761. Herbal remedies.

Neal's Yard Apothecary, 2 Neal's Yard, Covent Garden, London WC2. Tel. 01-379 7222.

PD **Sussex Herbs,** 9 Church Street, Seaford, E. Sussex BN25 1HD. Tel. Seaford (0323) 898914. Dried herbs and aromatherapy supplies. Mail order only – S.A.E. list.

PD **Taurbox Herbal Products,** Chitarras Manod Road, Blanau Ffestiniog, Gwynedd LL41 4AH. Tel. (0766) 831063. Suppliers of herbs. Bach flower remedies, essential and aromatic oils. 60p for catalogue and booklets.

PD **Witch Wood,** Oldfield Road, Bickley, Kent BR1 2LE. Aromatic oils, herbs, cosmetic kits, pot-pourri, bath preparations, shampoos. Mail order only – S.A.E. for price list.

As supplied with permission of magazine 'Herbal Review' Winter 1988.

Equivalents of Doses Used

1 Tablespoonful – ½ Fluid ounce
1 Wineglassful – 1½ -2 Fluid ounces
                or
                3-4 Tablespoonsful
1 Teacupful   – 4-5 Fluid ounces
                or
                8-10 Tablespoonsful

An Infusion is made by pouring 1 pint of boiling water over 1 ounce of the fresh herb or 1 teaspoonful of the dried herb, and allowing it to 'brew' for 5-10 minutes, before use.

A Decoction is made by boiling roots and/or seeds in water for 15-20 minutes, cooling and straining before use.

Condition: ABSCESS AND BOIL

DEFINITION
The white matter which fills an *abscess* and to a lesser extent a *boil* represents the dead leucocytes from the bloodstream, which have swallowed up bacteria invading the body and died. They also form a 'wall' blocking off the diseased area from other parts of the body to prevent the infection from spreading. An abscess or boil will tend to 'point' coming to the surface, discharging and leaving a crater-like ulcer.

CAUSE
(i)   Poor resistance to infections due to poor general health.

(ii)   Diet errors. Excess sugar in the diet is stored by the body in the tissues immediately below the skin, and if the skin is broken gives an excellent medium in which introduced infection can thrive.

SIGNS AND SYMPTOMS
(a)   Local redness, heat pain and swelling.

(b)   Body temperature may be raised.

(c)   There is a general feeling of 'not being well'.

TREATMENT
Treatment is divided into two groups:–

(A)   *Local treatment* at the point or area of infection.

(B)   *General treatment,* aimed to improve and maintain the body's resistance to infections.

(A) LOCAL TREATMENT
Consists of poulticing the area, to maintain the heat and moisture

which will encourage the abscess or boil to 'ripen' or 'point', as quickly as possible. Several *Poultices* are available:–

(i)   *Slippery Elm and Eucalyptus Oil*

Mix *Slippery Elm* powder with water to a thick consistency and add a few drops of *Eucalyptus Oil*. Spread the mixture on a piece of linen and apply the poultice to the affected area. Renew the poultice twice a day.

(ii)   *Linseed, Marshmallow and Oats*

Take two parts of *Linseed* powder, 1 part of *Marshmallow* dried and 1 part of *Oats* (crushed). Moisten these constituents with a soft paste of bread and milk.

Spread on a cloth and apply directly to the affected area.

Moisten with warm water periodically and renew at least twice a day.

(iii)   *Comfrey, Marshmallow, Plantain or Raspberry Leaves*

The leaves are crushed, dipped in hot water and applied.

(iv)   *Chickweed* Poultice. The *Chickweed* is used fresh, washed and applied directly. It is renewed every 6 hrs.

(B) GENERAL TREATMENT

Treatment in all cases must begin not only at the local area, but by building up the body's resistance. This is done by taking *Tonic Tisanes or Teas,* and attending to the *diet.*

(i)   *Agrimony Tea* or Tisane is an excellent starter. Take 1oz of the dried herb and on it pour 1 pint of boiling water. Allow it to brew or 'infuse' for 10 minutes. Take a teacupful 2 or 3 times a day. Sweetened with honey.

(ii)   ·*Coltsfoot Tea* has been handed down by the Romanies in a wonderful recipe as a 'cure' for all abscesses and sores. *Coltsfoot* leaves are boiled, and the '*Coltsfoot Tea*' is made so strong that when cold it sets into a jelly. It is eaten cold as a jelly or warmed and drunk as a tisane or tea.

(iii)   An excellent *tonic* handed down from folklore can be prepared as follows:–

Sweet Briar (Rose Hips) 3 parts

Black Currant (fruit) 1 part – by weight

Nettle (Leaves) 3 parts – by weight

Carrot (root) 3 parts

Add 1 tablespoonful of the mixture to 3 cupsful of boiling water. Allow to brew or infuse for 30 minutes., and take ½ teacupful 3 times a day.

DIET

Fresh Air and *Sunlight* in themselves are very good *tonics*.

Fish Liver Oils either *Cod* or *Halibut* either as an oil or in capsule form are needed at this time to give a good supply of the 'anti-infective factor' – vitamin A.

To build up the body's resistance, both silica rich and sulphur rich foods should be included in the diet. These include – raw cabbage, cucumber, lettuce, oatmeal and strawberries. Also figs, onions, oranges and radishes.

A liberal daily intake of *fresh fruit* and *salads* is indicated.

CONSULTANT OPINION

Consultant Herbalists would consider prescribing soothing poultices which would reduce the inflammation, be antiseptic and healing, by including the following herbs:–

(i)   *Marshmallow leaf* (Althaea officinalis) which is soothing, protective and heals wounds.

(ii)   *Linseed* (Linum usitatissimum) which has very soothing qualities.

(iii)   *Cone flower* (Echinacea augustifolia) which provides antiseptic and antiviral qualities.

(iv)   *Wood Sage* (Teucrium scorodonia) for healing wounds and destroying bacteria.

(v)   *Slippery Elm Bark* (Ulmus fulva) very soothing as a poultice and reducing inflammation.

Condition: ACNE

❀ ❀ ❀

DEFINITION

Acne is a skin disease which is very common in teenagers, but rarely arises after the age of 30 years. It is an inflammation of the hair and oil follicles in the skin and gives rise to blackheads, small solid red pimples, or pimples containing pus. In severe cases large painful nodules are formed, and in these areas scars may develop leaving permanent damage to the skin. The face, the back and the chest are the areas usually affected. Acne does not itch.

CAUSE

(i)   Excessive greasiness of the skin.

(ii)   Hormone changes in the individual taking place between the approximate ages of 14-25 yrs.

(iii) Digestive disorders. Over-indulgence in starchy and greasy foods in particular may aggravate the condition.

I recall an ancient couplet which goes:–

'If all goes right with the outside skin you may feel pretty sure all is right within' and of course the reverse often applies.

TREATMENT

Treatment is both *Local* at the site of the acne, and *General,* attending to 'internal' conditions and diet.

(A) LOCAL TREATMENT

(i)   Only use lukewarm water to wash the area.

(ii)   Avoid skin creams and powders. Two 'juices' can be used as a local 'wash':–

(i)   Diluted *Lemon Juice.* Dilute lemon juice with equal parts water as a skin wash.

(ii)   *Devilsbit Scabious Juice* has antiseptic as well as healing properties, and is a valuable skin wash.

(B) GENERAL TREATMENT

(a)   *Diet* is important. Meals should be supplemented with salads containing radishes, cress, watercress and dandelion leaves. Emphasis must be on avoiding too much sugar and tinned fatty foods. *Hormones* stabilise themselves naturally over a period of time, and this type of treatment is not interfered with, since this is normal development and growth.

(b)   The use of *tisanes* or *teas* is popular and always produces improvement if persevered with.

(i)   *Fumitory Tea.* Take 1oz of the fresh herb or 1 teaspoonful of the dried herb and to it add 1 pint of boiling water. Allow it to infuse (brew) for 10 minutes, and when cool take a wineglassful or 4 tablespoonsful every 3 hours.

(ii)   *Nettle Tea.* Make as for *Fumitory* tea (above) and take a similar dose, over a period of 2 weeks.

(iii) There is good report from a tisane of *Combined Herbs* as follows:–

Take equal parts (2ozs) of *Red Clover Flowers, Nettle Tops* and *Boneset.* Put the herbs into 2 quarts of boiling water and allow to simmer until reduced to 1 quart. When cool, add ginger or melted honey and take a wineglassful or 4 tablespoonsful every 3 hours.

To help to cure the digestive upsets common with this condition I know of two very helpful preparations.

The *first* has been given the name of 'Spring cleansing cure', and is a *tea* or *tisane.*

Take *Alder Buckthorn Bark* 3 parts
    Hartsease (violet) 3 parts
    Birch Leaves 2 parts
    Meadowsweet 2 parts

Mix well and add 1 tablespoonful of this mixture to 1 pint of boiling water, stand and strain. Drink one or two cupsful in the afternoon and evening.

The *second* is a decoction, prepared by *boiling* the herb in water for a period of 25-30 minutes. Take 1oz of *Burdock* – all parts of the plant can be used, and add 1½ pints of *cold* water. Bring to the boil, boil for ½ hour, cool and strain. Take 1 wineglassful or 4 tablespoonsful with every meal. This is an excellent remedy for skin eruptions of any kind.

CONSULTANT OPINION

A Consultant Herbalist might favour a specially prepared *herbal ointment* containing:–

(i)   *Poke Root* (Phytolacca decandra) which is a very popular anti-inflammatory agent.

(ii)   *Mountain Grape* (Berberis aquafolium) may also be used combined with *Yellow Dock Root* and *Burdock* in a herbal medicine in much use in treating skin conditions.

(iii)   *Golden Seal* (Hydrastis canadensis). Reduces inflammation and may be used in combination with *Witch Hazel* as a healing ointment.

Condition: ALOPECIA

❀ ❀ ❀

DEFINITION

Loss of Hair to some degree is very common. It affects roughly 4% of men and 10% of women. Several types of hair loss are known:–

(i)   *Common or male baldness*
(ii)   *General thinning of the hair*
(iii)   *Patchy loss of hair*
(iv)   *Total loss of hair*

The natural hair loss is rated at about 80 hairs per day. Each individual hair has a life of 2-5 years. The human being has more than a thousand hairs per square inch of scalp.

Each hair follicle rests for a while after it has shed a hair, and on the scalp about 90% of the follicles are active whilst 10% are resting.

(i)   *Common Male Baldness.* It is a normal accompaniment of advancing years, although it can occur prematurely before the age of 60 years, and even beginning in the 20s. There is a thinning or absence of hair from around the top of the head, with a recession of the margins in front.

(ii)   *General thinning of the hair* can occur in any of these conditions:–

(a)   Following an acute fever, e.g. influenza.
(b)   After childbirth.
(c)   Alongside debilitating illness such as diabetes.
(d)   Tuberculosis.
(e)   Anaemia.

When the general health improves so does the condition of the hair.

(iii)   *Patchy Loss of Hair.* Known as alopecia. Each 'patch' is clear cut, smooth and shiny, with normal hair growth surrounding it.

(iv)   *Total loss of hair.* Known as *total alopecia* and is a more severe condition than the one described above.

See *'Ringworm'* for patchy hair loss in children.

CAUSES
1.   A *Hereditary factor* in common baldness following the tendency in father and grandfather.
2.   *Male sex hormone* which stimulates the secretion of scalp oil associated with hair loss. A good head of hair is as characteristic of the eunuch as the absence of beard.
3.   Women tend to suffer from 'thinning' after the menopause when female hormone production has ebbed.
4.   Patchy baldness or alopecia has been associated with *psychological or nervous debility.*

TREATMENT

It is considered that the process of 'balding' can be hindered or even halted. Treatment is either *Local* and/or *General*.

(A) LOCAL TREATMENT

(i)   One of the traditional hair restorers is *Yarrow*.

Prepare a tisane, take 1oz of the herb fresh or 1 teaspoonful of the dried herb, pour on 1 pint of boiling water. Cool and rub the liquid on the scalp. Indeed, this prepared tea can be taken as a medicine in a dose of a wineglassful or 4 tablespoonsful.

(ii)   *Nettle Juice* extracted with a juicer is said to stimulate the growth of hair on the scalp. Dilute the juice with water using 1 teaspoonful of the juice to a cup of water. Experiment with the strength for individual application.

(iii)   A very ancient recipe used since the time of the Pharoahs in Egypt, is to boil *Willow Leaves* in oil – modern vegetable oil will do, and place the leaves on the bald or thin areas.

(iv)   *Coconut Oil* rubbed on the scalp has wide application in Eastern Countries.

(v)   The herb *Rosemary* is the one of choice, it is said to have a tonic action and will prevent premature balding.

'*Rosemary Brew*' is made by taking 2 or 3 sprigs of *Rosemary*, (both twigs and leaves), breaking them up into ½ pint of cold water, bringing this to the boil and simmering for 3 minutes. The brew should be left to stand overnight, stored in a jar – earthenware if possible – and should be massaged into the head 3 or 4 times a week. The longer the brew is kept the stronger it becomes. Never drain it. It can be used as a 'Setting Lotion'.

(B) GENERAL TREATMENT

(i)   Patchy hair loss is considered to be associated with nervous debility, therefore it is advisable to take a nerve tonic and restorative to restore good health.

The following prescription is to be recommended:–

Take *1 part* each of the following herbs:–

Valerian Root, Peppermint Leaves, Chamomile Flowers, Caraway Seed and Fennel Seed. Take 1 tablespoonful of this mixture, place it in cold water, bring to the boil, allow it to stand for 15-20 minutes. Take ½ cupful each morning and evening.

(ii) If there is thinning of the hair associated with debilitating illness, a fresh fruit, raw vegetable diet is advised with a high vitamin intake daily.

CONSULTANT OPINION

Local treatment by Consultant Herbalists is purely speculative and individual.

(i)   *Tincture of Arnica* B.P.C. has been recommended for external application in alopecia, but this remedy is poorly tolerated by some people. It must only be applied to unbroken skin, and withdrawn on the first sign of skin irritation.

General Treatment by the Consultant consists usually of a good nerve tonic and restorative and may contain such herbs as:–

(i)   *Kola Nuts* (Cola nitida) which is a stimulant to the nervous system, improving the mood and appetite.

(ii)   *Saw Palmetto* (Serenoa serrulata) which corrects loss of weight and general debility after illness.

(iii)   *Damiana* (Turnera diffusa) which improves the mood and the sense of well being.

Condition: ANAEMIA

DESCRIPTION

Simple Anaemia means a lower than normal concentration of the iron-containing red pigment in the blood called haemoglobin. Haemoglobin conveys oxygen in the circulation to the brain, muscles and other organs and lack of it gives rise to the characteristic 'symptoms of anaemia'.

CAUSES

(i)   Loss of blood from severe bleeding.

(ii)   A slow loss over a period of time from heavy menstrual bleeding or bleeding piles.

(iii)   Incorrect diet with lack of the normal blood forming constituents – iron, trace elements, and Vitamin B12.

(iv)   General illnesses such as rheumatoid arthritis.

SIGNS AND SYMPTOMS

These include pallor of the skin, weakness, giddiness, rapid breathing and palpitation of the heart, breathlessness on exertion and sore tongue. There is also a lack of energy, cold hands and feet and sometimes a feeling of anxiety. All ages can be affected, the young being more prone than the elderly, and it is not confined to any one sex.

TREATMENT

(A) *Fresh air, adequate rest* and *exercise in moderation* are all advised.

(B) *Diet* must be nutritious and of a kind containing the blood forming elements and those rich in iron. These include:– liver, kidney, beef, herrings, dried fruit and vegetables, spinach, lettuce, peas, watercress, eggs, marmite, bovril, treacle and breakfast oats. Spinach juice and carrot juice have found favouritism with the Romanies. They are readily available with the juice extractor.

(C) *Tisanes or Teas* have an important placing in treating simple anaemia.

(i) *Centaury Tea* this tisane is a 'must' in the treatment of debility and anaemia. Use 1oz of fresh *Centaury* or 1 teaspoonful of the dried herb to 1 pint of boiling water. Allow to brew (infuse) for 10 minutes then take a wineglassful or 4 tablespoonsful three times a day.

(ii) An excellent remedy for a simple anaemia is a *'decoction'* of 4 herbs. Here the herbs are 'boiled'.

Take *Yellow Dock* ¹/₂oz

    Bogbean ¹/₂oz

    Agrimony ¹/₂oz

    Marshmallow Leaves 1oz

Boil in 2 quarts of water until this is reduced to 1 quart. Take a wineglassful or 4 tablespoonsful 3 times a day after allowing it to cool and straining it.

(iii) The 'anaemia' herbs *Bogbean, Clivers, Fumitory* and *Senna* can all be boiled together, taking ¹/₂oz of each in 2 pints of water and boiling until the volume is reduced to 1 pint. The resulting cooled and strained liquid is taken in doses of 1 wineglassful or 4 tablespoonsful 3 times a day.

(iv) *Nettle* Tisane. Using 1oz of the fresh herb or 1 teaspoonful of the dried herb to 1 pint of boiling water and infusing for 10 minutes gives a pleasant restorative for anaemia subjects if sweetened with honey.

The dose is a wineglassful or 4 tablespoonsful 3 times a day.
We maintain that herbal cures are slow but sure and treatments for simple anaemia should continue for a least a month. A simple anaemia once diagnosed as such will respond quite readily to herbal therapy. If the response is unsatisfactory, further investigations are advised, and a visit to the doctor.

CONSULTANT OPINION
(i)   *Iron* in the form of *Ferrous Gluconate* tablets can be taken over a period of months. 'Anaemic Herbs' used by the Consultant include:–
(ii)   *Agrimony* (Agrimonia eupatoria) a 'tonic'.
(iii)   *Greater Periwinkle* (Vinca major) a blood 'purifier'.
(iv)   *Cone Flower* (Echinacea augustifolia) a 'stimulant' to good circulation.
(v)   *Hops* (Avena sativa) improves the mood relieves attendant depression.
(vi)   *Poke Root* (Phytolacca decandra) a blood 'purifier'.
(vii)   *Saw Palmetto Berries* (Serenea serrulata) improves the general body condition.

Condition: BRONCHIAL ASTHMA

DEFINITION
Bronchial Asthma is a sudden temporary attack of difficult breathing with a sense of suffocation, and difficulty in breathing out.

CAUSE
(i)   An *allergic* element, frequently household dusts.
(ii)   A *stress* factor.

SIGNS AND SYMPTOMS
The attacks frequently arise in the early hours of the morning around 2 or 3 a.m. The patient is acutely distressed with tightness across the chest and difficulty in breathing. There is 'wheezing' and a sense of suffocation.
All this is accompanied by heavy sweating. By morning the symptoms tend to abate.

TREATMENT

Treatment is initially directed towards removing the suffocating tightness of the chest and sedating the irritating non-productive cough. *Tisanes* or *Teas* are prepared from either *single* herbs or *compound mixtures* of herbs:–

(i)   *Ephedra* Tea. *Ephedra* or ma-juang contains a special ingredient which opens the airways in the chest when taken. It can be bought in some Chinese shops in Great Britain.

It is prepared by using 1oz of the whole herb, pouring on 1 pint of boiling water, allowing it to brew or infuse for 10 minutes, and taking the 'tea' in doses of a wineglassful or 4 tablespoonsful 3 or 4 times a day.

(ii)   *German Chamomile* or *Matricaria*, is a favourite with childhood asthmas.

Take 6 flower heads of *Chamomile* and infuse them with 1 pint of boiling water. Tablespoonful doses are advised.

(iii)   *Euphorbia Herb* tea is noted for its relief of chest tightness. Infuse 1oz of the herb with a pint of boiling water. Tablespoonful doses should be given.

(iv)   Asthma sufferers almost always benefit by drinking a cup of *strong coffee* without sugar or milk.

(v)   A *mixture of herbs* from which children derive much benefit is prepared as follows:–

Take *Coltsfoot* 2 parts

        White *Horehound* 2 parts

Take 5 teaspoonsful of the mixed herbs and infuse with 3 cupsful of boiling water for 20 minutes, strain, add honey to sweeten and give a dose of 1-4 tablespoonsful 4 times a day depending upon the age of the child.

(vi)   Take *equal parts* of crushed *Aniseed, Liquorice* root, *Plantain* leaves, *Fennel* seed and *Coltsfoot* leaves. Infuse 1 teaspoonful of the mixed herbs with ½ cup boiling water for 10 minutes, strain, sweeten with honey or brown sugar, and take ½ teacupful 3 times a day.

(vii)   Take *equal* parts of *Marshmallow* leaves and flowers, mull flowers and leaves, *Coltsfoot* leaves and *Liquorice* root. Thoroughly mix all ingredients and infuse 1 teaspoonful of the mixed herbs with ½ cup boiling water for 10 minutes, strain, sweeten and take ½ teacupful 3 times a day.

CONSULTANT OPINION

The Consultant Herbalist has a very wide variety of herbs to choose from in preparing his mixtures of tinctures to treat asthma.

Some of these would perhaps be combinations as follows:–

(i)   *Ephedra* combined with *Lobelia, Grindelia* and *Skunkweed*

or

(ii)   *Drosera* (Sundew) combined with *Euphorbia, Grindelia* or *Senaga*

or

(iii)   *Blood Root* combined with *Lobelia.*

Many more combinations of herbs could be used to great advantage, such as:–

(iv)   *Snake Root* with *Euphorbia* and *Grindelia*

or

(v)   *Squills* with *Horehound* and *Coltsfoot.*

Condition: BEDWETTING OR ENURESIS

DEFINITION

The term *Bedwetting* explains itself. In the medical world it is called *Enuresis,* and it refers to the inability of the young child to 'control' the bladder function during its early years.

We use the term *Nocturnal Enuresis* when there is no control during the night hours, but when this disability extends to the daytime also we call it *Diurnal* enuresis.

The average age at which an infant is 'dry' during the *daytime* is 2-3 years, but night control usually extends to 3-5 years or even above this age. For another year we might still consider it to be within normal limits.

A child in its early years can sometimes return to wetting the bed after a period of 'dryness', and very rarely in the 'relapsed' cases do we expect them to be dry again before the age of 7 years.

CAUSES

(1)   Bedwetting in a child who has never been dry, we call *primary enuresis,* and in these cases we must consider a *hereditary* factor. This

type of bedwetting should not concern us unduly, as it will eventually clear up.

(ii)   The child may have a *small bladder* which is unable to hold a great deal. Boys are known to have smaller bladders than girls. Very rarely do we find a malformation.

(iii)   'Emotional' factors must be considered in dealing with a child who returns to bedwetting after a long dry period. *Jealousy, excessive strictness, bullying* at school, or having to *go into hospital* could be the cause.

(iv)   On the other hand, childhood fevers or infections in the urinary tract itself could be the cause of such a relapse.

TREATMENT

(a)   In the normal average child, encouraging it to 'wait a little longer' by day, will help it to gain some control and the bladder itself will slowly grow to hold more.

(b)   It is imperative that all 'physical' causes of bedwetting should be removed before attempting any routine.

(c)   'Dryness' should be rewarded, but on the other hand there should be no punishment for failures.

(d)   A child should have essential security, love and understanding to promote its development along right lines.

(e)   Bedwetters have been found to have a deficiency of both *Silicon* and *Calcium* in their bodies, and two herbs go a long way to helping to relieve this:–

(i)   *Horsetail Grass* Tisane:– use 1 teaspoonful to 1 pint of boiling water. Allow it to brew, and take doses of a wineglassful – 4 tablespoonsful of the tea.

(ii)   *Thyme* tea is made as above using 1 teaspoonful of dried thyme to the pint of boiling water.

Should the bedwetting be found to be aggravated by threadworms an excellent treatment is to use the thyme tea sweetened with honey, but make the tea or tisane much stronger, using 3 teaspoonsful of the dried herb to a pint of water.

CONSULTANT OPINION

Herbs available to Consultant Herbalists and used in their preparations as either Tinctures or Liquid Extracts include:–

(i)   *Corn Silk* (Zea Mays) – valuable if there is inflammation in the urinary tract.

(ii)   *Horsetail Grass* (Equisetum arvense) – a herb which reduces local inflammation and discharge.

(iii)   *Cramp Bark* (Viburnum opulus) is very soothing and reduces any tendency to spasm or muscular cramps.

(iv)   *Thyme* (Thymus vulgaris) known to arrest the growth of bacteria. It also relaxes muscle cramps.

(v)   *Greater Periwinkle* (Vinca major) well known as reducing inflammation.

Treatment is directed towards reducing the possibility of any infection and preventing complications.

Condition: BITES AND STINGS

❀ ❀ ❀

DESCRIPTION

A *Bite* is described as a wound or puncture made by the mouth parts of a living organism.

A *Sting* is injury caused by the venom of a plant or animal where poison is introduced.

All *natural* kingdoms are involved – *Insect, Plant,* and *Animal,* by far the largest being the *insects.*

Common *Insects* which sting or bite include gnats, mosquitoes, bees, wasps, hornets, fleas and tics.

The most common offender in the *Plant* kingdom is the stinging-nettle which is covered with fine stiff hairs which penetrate the skin. The only native *Animal* (Reptile) which injects venom into its bite is the viper or adder, and this is only very rarely. Amongst the *insects* the bee is also unwilling to sting unless severely provoked, as the barbs of the sting, once inserted, cannot be withdrawn, and the bee dies.

PREVENTION

Herbal preparations are used to *repel* insects. The Romanies are very wise in this respect, and the repellent commonly used in the countryside is *Feverfew* or Bachelor Buttons.

A few leaves are collected, a pint of boiling water is poured over them, and the infusion is left for about 10 minutes. The lotion is allowed to cool and is then sponged on the skin and allowed to dry. This is an excellent 'preventative' for the bites of gnats and mosquitoes.

Other *repellents* include the volatile *Oil* of *Lavender, Citronella Eucalyptus* and *Sassafras.*

Oily skins are not always acceptable and as these oils carry a heavy smell they are not very popular.

TREATMENT

(i)   For *Gnat Bites* and *Mosquito Bites* first aid treatment to immediately stop the itching is to dab on damp salt in small lumps. The spots quickly disappear also.

(ii)   *Vinegar* too is effective if dabbed on and allowed to dry.

(iii)   *Bee and Wasp Stings* or stings by other 'venomous' insect such as the Hornet can be treated with raw *Onion.* Just rub it on the area, or bandage slices of onion on.

(iv)   *Witch Hazel* is a powerful antiseptic and very useful for *Wasp* stings. Dab on the lotion.

(v)   In trying to prevent *fleabites,* clothes should be washed in water containing either *Wormwood* or *Fleabane, Chamomile* and *Alder* are also helpful.

(vi)   For other serious bites such as a *dog bite* a poultice of *Fennel Seeds* 'draws out' any poison and infection.

(vii)   *Snake Bites* are potentially more dangerous. The only poisonous snake native to these shores is the Viper or Adder. This snake is usually quite harmless, and normally will only bite if frightened or trodden on.

Most *Snake Bites* destroy some constituents of the blood, and many affect the nervous system within a very short interval of time – say around 15 minutes. The *victim* becomes *faint,* has *difficulty* in *breathing* and may quickly become *paralysed.*

SNAKE BITES

Immediate treatment is to place a tight band above the bite, and if necessary a cut should be made over the wound about 1 inch long, and $\frac{1}{2}$" deep, press, wash and suck the wound. Any sucked out material must be spat out immediately.

Seek *professional advice immediately.*

Basil crushed and applied directly on the bites of venomous insects or snakes has a value, so have *Honeysuckle* leaves and leaves of *Devils Bit* and *Vipers Bugloss.*

An *antidote* to the bites of *venomous creatures* is said to be *Honeysuckle Tea* using 1oz of the dried leaves to 1 pint of boiling water, infuse for 10 minutes and take in wineglassful doses, whilst rubbing the hands with the juice of *radishes* is a powerful repellent.

Plant Stings are not considered to be so obnoxious, and nettle stings are adequately dealt with by rubbing *Dock, Plantain, Elder* or *Horseradish* leaves on the affected area.

Vinegar too is effective, and in season the cool white fur of the inside of the pod of the *Broad Bean*. This is very soothing.

Some plants however produce *allergic* skin reactions when they come in contact with the skin, and a *tisane* or *tea* of a combination of herbs is very helpful. Take 1 pinch of each of the following herbs – *Basil, Rosemary, Thyme, Vervain* and *Aniseed*. Add 2 cups of boiling water, leave for 10 minutes, and take wineglassful doses.

Condition: BLOOD PRESSURE

DESCRIPTION

Blood Pressure is the pressure of the circulating blood on the walls of the blood vessels which contain it. The normal rise and fall coincides with the rise and fall in the pumping action of the heart creating the heartbeat.

Blood Pressure is taken in the brachial artery of the arm. The highest blood pressure is that which is required to obliterate the pulse at the wrist. This is called the *systolic pressure*. In the young adult the normal systolic blood pressure reads 100-120mm on the sphygmomanometer or blood pressure apparatus.

The *diastolic* pressure or lowest pressure is the normal pressure in the artery in the resting phase of the heartbeat, and in the young adult the reading is 70-90mm.

CAUSES

An increase in the Blood Pressure above normal can be due to an increase in physical effort, stress or emotional factors, or it can be due to a 'hardening of the arteries' or arteriosclerosis, and some kinds of kidney disease, or heart disease. It is called *Hypertension*.

Hypotension, or an abnormally low blood pressure may be caused by shock, or diseases of the circulation. Therefore it is of paramount importance that persistent changes from the normal average levels of blood pressure should be known to the doctor and kept under observation and supervision. The doctor should be in full knowledge of any subsidiary herbal therapies.

SIGNS AND SYMPTOMS
Symptoms of *unacceptable variations* in blood pressure include:– Headaches, giddiness, 'walking-on-air', depression, insomnia, noises in the head and ears, a 'muddled' head and general irritability.

TREATMENT
Practically all the following plants produce only a *temporary* lowering of blood pressure. Treatment must be continued for a long time.

Extracts from some plants, both *tropical* and *indigenous* (native) have yielded very active drugs which are used to lower blood pressure, but they must only be taken under medical supervision. They include *Rao wolfia* and *White Hellebore.*

Amongst our native plants we include *Garlic, Ransomes, Hawthorn* and *Artichoke.* If the blood pressure is *low,* however, *Ginseng* tea and *Rosemary* tea have a place in treatment.

TREATMENT OF HIGH BLOOD PRESSURE
(i)   *Garlic.* Using the *fresh* plant, finely slice or crush 1 fresh garlic clove. Spread on bread or mix in lukewarm milk. Take 1 clove 2-3 times daily for several months.

or

(ii)   *Garlic Juice.* Press 2-3 fresh garlic cloves. Drink mixed with warm milk or in honey. Take 2-3 times daily for several months.

(iii)   *Artichoke.* To make a tisane pour 1 cup of cold water over 1-2 teaspoonsful of dried leaves. Bring to the boil and let boil for 1 minute. Let stand for 5-10 minutes. Take 1 cup 2-3 times daily for a week or longer.

(iv)   *Hawthorn Tea.* Pour 1 cup boiling water over 2 teaspoonsful of blossoms or leaves. Let stand for 20 minutes. Take 1 cup 2-3 times daily.

(v)   For *Chair-bound Obese people* who suffer from hypertension a simple tisane of *nettles* is recommended:–

Boil 1oz of common nettles with 1 pint of water for 10 minutes. Take 2 tablespoonsful 2-3 times a day.

(vi)　*Burdock Root.* Rich in iron helps to combat any anaemia. Use crushed and sliced root, and simmer 1oz of the root with $^1/_3$ pint water. Simmer for 15 minutes, allow to steep, then drink $^1/_2$ cupful, warmed and sweetened with honey. In the kitchen *Chives* helps to keep the blood pressure down. Use them in omlettes, soups and vegetable broths. Chopped chives in butter and spread on grilled steak is delicious.

TREATMENT OF LOW BLOOD PRESSURE

(i)　*Ginseng* has acquired a good reputation, taken either in the prepared tablet form, purchased from our Health Stores or a *Ginseng Tea,* which can be prepared by adding 1 cup of water to $^1/_2$ teaspoonful of the shredded root. Boil for 1 minute, let stand for 15 minutes, then take a cupful twice daily.

(ii)　*Rosemary Tea.* Use 1 cup of boiling water to 1 teaspoonful of fresh or dried leaves, let stand for 20 minutes. Take a cupful twice daily.

For the *'regulation'* of blood pressure, i.e. maintaining it at a healthy level, I would suggest:–

(i)　Eat *Garlic.*

(ii)　Drink infusions of *Hawthorn Tea.*

(iii)　Make up the following herbal infusion using *multiple herbs:–*

Take a *pinch* of each of the following:– *Mint, Basil, Vervain,* and *Chamomile,* infuse with 1 pint of boiling water. Stand for 10 minutes then take a large cupful every night.

CONSULTANT OPINION

In the treatment of *Hypertension* (High Blood Pressure) the Consultant Herbalist might choose to use one or other of the following herbs:–

(i)　*Hawthorn Berries* (Crataegus monogyna). The special indications are where there is hypertension with heart pain or angina, or the heart muscle itself is weak, and it is used in combination with *Night Blooming Cereus, Thyme Flowers, Mistletoe* or *Skullcap.*

(ii)　*Buckwheat* (Fagopyrum esculentum). It is used in cases of hypertension with bleeding in the smallest blood vessels, i.e. capillaries.

(iii)　*Yarrow* (Achillea millefolium), is used combined with *Lime Flowers* in the condition of thrombosis, i.e. clots forming in the blood vessels.

(iv)   *Lime Flowers* (Tilia platyphyllos), very valuable in treating 'hardening of the arteries'.

(v)   *Mistletoe* (Viscum album) whose specific indication for use is in raised blood pressure.

In the treatment of *Hypotension,* i.e. low blood pressure, the treatment might include:–

(i)   *Ginseng* (Panax schinseng). Valuable in glandular weakness in the body.

or

(ii)   *Broom Tops* (Sarothamnus scoparius). The specific indication for the use of broom tops is where there is present palpitations, with weakness of the heart muscle. It is advisable not to take broom tops during pregnancy.

Condition: BRONCHITIS

❀ ❀ ❀

DEFINITION

Bronchitis is inflammation of the bronchial tubes. The windpipe or trachea, forks into two in the upper chest, and each individual branch is called a *Bronchus,* and leads directly to the lungs.

CAUSES

(i)   Colds and chills.

(ii)   Undue exposure to the elements.

(iii)   Inhaling irritant substances.

(iv)   The aftermath of chest infections such as influenza.

SIGNS AND SYMPTOMS

(a)   Fever – if the cause is an infection.

(b)   Chest pain on coughing.

(c)   Breathlessness.

(d)   Coughing which does not produce sputum in the early stages.

(e)   Coughing which produces profuse muco-purulent sputum or phlegm in the later stages, and represents the discarded lining of the bronchi.

TREATMENT

(A)   To ease a Hard Dry Cough, bring down fever and promote perspiration take the following 'first-aid' therapies.

(i)   An *Elderberry, Peppermint and Composition Mixture* (known as E.P.C.) available at all good Health Stores. Take the dose according to instructions on the bottle.

The essential herbal constituents of this mixture are *Elderberry Flowers, Peppermint* and a *Composition Essence* which includes *Bayberry, Hemlock Spruce, Capsicum, Cassia, Clove* and *Pimento Oils.*

(ii)   A *home-made brew or tisane.* Take *equal parts* of the following herbs – *Liquorice Root, Coltsfoot Flowers, Mallow Flowers, Thyme* and *Crushed Aniseed.* Take 2 tablespoonsful of the mixed herbs and on it pour $^1\!/_2$ pint of boiling water. Allow it to brew for 10 minutes. Sweeten with honey, add Rum or Brandy if desired and take a wineglassful or 4 tablespoonsful two or three times a day.

(B)   To relieve the 'dryness' and tightness of the chest, Poulticing should follow.

Poulticing improves local circulation, removes toxins or poisons from the area, and since poultices contain healing herbal oils, these can be readily absorbed through the skin surface.

Poulticing should be carried out on both the front and the back of the chest. Two popular poultices for this purpose are (a) *Kaolin Poultice* – obtained from any chemist. It has a china clay base to retain the heat, and oil of *Wintergreen* is the healing oil which is incorporated. The *Kaolin* is heated, spread on a cloth, and applied directly to the skin area.

(b)   *Linseed Poultice.* Which is 'home-made'. Add 9ozs of *Linseed flour* to $1^3\!/_4$ pints of boiling water. It is further boiled to thicken it. Add a pinch of *Wild Thyme* and *Mint*, or sprinkle the surface with powdered *Ginger*. Renew the poultice every 12 hours. Poultices are very soothing.

(C)   When the feverish coughing stage has passed, encourage coughing to produce the phlegm of the 'catarrh'.

This 'clearing of the chest' is completed by taking herbal tisanes or teas.

(a)   A *'combined'* tisane of *Marshmallow, Linseed* and *Liquorice.*

Take *Marshmallow leaves* 1 part

    Linseed 2 parts

    Liquorice 1 part

Mix thoroughly.

To 1 teaspoonful of the mixture add ½ teacupful of boiling water. Allow to brew for 10 minutes, then take ½ teacupful 2 or 3 times a day and as hot as possible.

(b)   A tisane of *equal* parts of:–

Elecampane Root, Thyme, Nettle leaves and *Lungwort*. Mix the herbs together thoroughly then take 1 teaspoonful to 1 teacupful of boiling water. Brew for 10 minutes and take ½ teacupful 2 or 3 times a day.

(c)   A 'chest' prescription which has stood the test of time consists of:–

Marshmallow Root 2 teaspoonsful

Liquorice 2 teaspoonsful

Golden Seal 2 teaspoonsful

Pleurist Root 2 teaspoonsful

Linseed ½oz

Icelandic Moss ½oz

Place the herbs in a *quart* of cold water, boil for 5 minutes occasionally stirring, strain whilst hot, add 2ozs of sugar.

Allow the mixture to cool, and only take it when *cold* in a wineglassful or 4 tablespoonful doses, 2 or 3 times a day.

(d)   A favourite prescription is:–

Take *1oz* of each of the following 6 herbs:–

White Horehound, Hyssop, Vervain, Agrimony, Bogbean and *Liquorice Root.* Add 2 quarts of water. Reduce to ½ quantity by boiling and take a wineglassful or 4 tablespoonsful 3 times a day.

CONSULTANT OPINION

The Consultant Herbalist uses *Tinctures* and *Liquid Extracts* of Herbs in preparing prescriptions. These are prepared according to strict, accurate standards of efficiency, and are available only to members of the profession.

In treating *Bronchitis,* the following herbs could be dispensed:–

(i)   *Garlic* (Allium sativum). It is antiseptic, inhibits the further growth of bacteria, produces sweating and encourages the production of sputum.

(ii)   *Angelica* (Angelica archangelica) reduces 'tightness' in the chest and encourages the production of phlegm.

(iii)   *Elecampane Root* (Inula helenium). Relieves the irritating cough of children and catarrh.

(iv)   *Lungwort* (Pulmonia officinalis). Soothing to the bronchial tubes and encouraging the 'loose' cough which gets rid of phlegm.

(v)   *Coltsfoot* (Tussilago farfara). Valuable in treatment in the early stages of bronchitis to ease an irritable cough.

(vi) *Mullein* (Verbascum thapsus). Soothing, healing, and encouraging the production of sputum to 'clear' the bronchial tubes.

There are many others of popular choice.

Condition: BRUISES

❀ ❀ ❀

DESCRIPTION

A *bruise* is a superficial injury produced by an impact without producing a torn or ragged wound, but resulting in local haemorrhage.

SIGNS AND SYMPTOMS TREATMENT

(1) *Pain.*   (2) *Swelling.*   (3) *Local Discoloration* of the area.

Treatment is in the main by *Compresses* of various *individual* herbs, or *combined* herbs.

(a)   *Marigold Compress.* Pour a pint of boiling water over 2 teaspoonsful of chopped *Marigold Herb.* Leave for 10 minutes, then make a cool compress to cover the bruised area. Apply the compress frequently.

(b)   *Witch Hazel Compress.* Add 1 pint of cold water to 2 teaspoonsful of the leaves and bark of the *Witch Hazel* Shrub. Boil for 15 minutes, let it stand for 15 minutes. Strain and make a cool compress. Change frequently and do not allow the compress to dry out.

(c)   *Melilot Compress.* Add 1 pint of cold water to 2 tablespoonsful of the fresh or dried herb. Boil for 1 minute. Stand for 20 minutes. Strain and use as a cool compress. Apply frequently.

To reduce pain and swelling, a simple soothing *ointment* can be made in the home by taking *nettle* leaves, bruising them, mixing them with both *salt* and *Malt vinegar* and incorporating this in a lard base.

(d)   A confirmed favourite prescription using *combined herbs* in a *compress* is known as the *'Wiltshire Preparation'.* Take an autumn or spring root of *Comfrey,* scrubbed clean and steep this in a jar of *Witch Hazel* lotion from the chemist.

Keep the preparation in a warm place for several weeks. Strain the liquid, store it and use it as the occasion arises as a cold compress.

Certain herbs have specific healing properties for different areas of the body, e.g. the 'Black Eye'. Similar healing properties for bruising around the eye are found in (a) *Hyssop Leaves* and (b) *Purple Loosestrife*. *Hyssop Leaves* or *Purple Loosestrife Leaves* are tied in a linen bag, soaked in boiling water, allowed to cool sufficiently, then held over the bruised area around the eye.

The *discoloration* of bruising can quickly be removed in any area by mixing a 'paste' of pounded *Marjoram Leaves* with *Honey* and applying the paste to the bruised area.

If bruising has been *severe,* several herbs help to bring about the reabsorption of the local haemorrhage, and to this end a *Poultice* of *Sassafras, Comfrey, Rowan, Chamomile* and *Figwort* in a suitable base such as *Slippery Elm Bark* powder or *Linseed* flour is prepared. Pain and swelling are quickly reduced.

The following tisane or tea helps the reabsorption of bruising.

Take *Shepherd's Purse* 3 parts
  Lady's Mantle 3 parts
  Silverweed 2 parts
  Woodruff 2 parts

Take 1 tablespoonful of the *mixed* herbs and on it pour ½ pint of boiling water. Cover and allow to stand for 10 minutes.

Drink a cupful between each meal and eat as little sweet food as possible.

Condition: NASAL CATARRH AND SINUSITIS

DEFINITION

Nasal Catarrh is an inflammation of the mucous membrane which lines the canals and cavities of the nose, throat and ears which communicate with the outside, and produces a constant state of 'stuffiness' or discharge from the nose itself.

The term 'catarrh' is frequently applied to a head cold which fails to clear up.

CAUSE

(i)   Infection which does not clear.

(ii)   'Catarrh' sufferers belong to one of two classes of individual:–

(a)   *Class I* – does not like exercise, fresh air or excitement. They are fond of food perhaps a little too much, artificial warmth, hot baths and many clothes. The nose is permanently blocked, or dripping profusely down the back of the throat.

(b)   *Class II* – Eager, 'keyed-up' individuals always 'on the ball'.

SIGNS AND SYMPTOMS

(i)   There can be free discharge of mucus and pus from the nose.

(ii)   Headaches.

(iii)   Sometimes stuffiness in the nose encourages mouth breathing.

(iv)   There is a general feeling of being 'below the weather'.

If the hollow air-spaces in the cheek-bones and behind the eyebrows become inflamed, because of the structure of these spaces, infected material cannot easily drain away and a condition known as *Sinusitis* arises.

Factors which can worsen catarrh in both class I and class II individuals, include:–

(a)   *The use of nasal drops and sprays* which become habit forming and turn a temporary relief to a permanent disability.

(b)   Smoking is irritating.

(c)   Alcohol causes further congestion.

(d)   Anxieties over such things as home, work, money and children.

TREATMENT

(i)   Revolutionise your way of life whether you belong to class I or class II.

(ii)   Instead of using nasal drops and nasal sprays try inhalations of the following:–

(a)   *Eucalyptus Steam.* Use 1 teaspoonful of *Eucalyptus Oil* to a pint of boiling water. Inhale the steam along with the eucalyptus vapour.

(b)   *Olbas Oil* is a blend of pure plant oils including *Cajuput Oil B.P.C., Clove Oil B.P., Eucalyptus Oil B.P., Juniper Berry Oil, Menthol B.P., Peppermint Oil B.P.* and *Wintergreen Oil P.P.C.*

Inhalations of *Olbas Oil* clear nasal congestion caused by colds, bronchial catarrh, influenza and sinusitis.

(iii)   Take *Garlic* daily whether in tablet or capsule form. Garlic will eventually bring about a cure, if not immediately, will do so in weeks, provided the treatment is continued.

(iv)   Take *Lemon Juice* and *Honey* as often as desired.

(v)   Serve *Sage Tea* with lemon juice instead of milk and sweetened with a little honey. The sage tea is prepared using a teaspoonful of dried sage to a pint of boiling water, allowing it to brew for 10 minutes before use.

(vi)   A tisane of a compound mixture of herbs is very useful.

Take equal parts of *Elder Flowers, Peppermint* and *Yarrow*. Use 1 teaspoonful of the mixture to a pint of boiling water. The dose is a wineglassful or 4 tablespoonsful 3 times a day.

or

(vii)   Take *Coltsfoot* ½oz, *Mullein* 1oz, *Sage* 1oz, *Thyme* 2oz, *Yarrow* 2ozs. Mix the herbs thoroughly and put them into a quart of water. Bring to the boil and simmer until it is reduced to half the quantity. Take a wineglassful or 4 tablespoonsful 3 times a day, until the catarrh clears.

Diet is important in treating 'catarrh'.

(a)   Rich starchy foods should be avoided such as potatoes, pastries, chocolates, sweets and cakes.

'Unhelpful' vegetables include haricot beans, preserved peas, and woody turnips.

To build up the general health, *vitamin rich vegetables* should be taken such as Brussels sprouts, cabbage, carrots, white turnip, runner beans, young fresh peas, and spinach. *Fresh salads* including celery, tomatoes, and radishes are said to give antiseptic protection.

CONSULTANT OPINION

Some of the popular herbs used by the Consultant Herbalist in prescribing treatment for catarrh and sinusitis include:–

(i)   *Althaea Leaf* (Althaea officinalis). It soothes and protects the lining membrane of the nose and throat.

(ii)   *Wild Indigo* (Baptisia tinctoria). It is germicidal and antiseptic. It also promotes sweating, to rid the body of its poisons.

(iii)   *Poke Root* (Phytolacca decandra). It eases pain and reduces the tendency for the mucus membrane to become catarrhal.

(iv)   *Lungwort* (Pulmonaria officinalis) is soothing and reduces the inflammation.

(v)   *Marsh Cudweed* (Gnaphalium uliginosum) gives an antiseptic element preventing catarrh.

(vi)   *Golden Rod* (Solidago virgaurea) is antiseptic, promotes sweating and is popular as a gargle in nose and throat infections.

Condition: CHILBLAINS

❀ ❀ ❀

DEFINITION

Chilblains are dusky red, oval swellings occurring on the fingers, feet, and occasionally on the tips of the ears and the nose. They are itchy or intensely irritating. They can become transparent blisters which break, leaving ulcerated areas. Broken chilblains are very painful and difficult to heal.

CAUSES

(i)   A sudden lowering of *outside temperature* plus *dampness*. These climatic conditions can give rise to an exaggerated response by the blood vessels in the areas concerned.

(ii)   A *deficiency* of *calcium* and *silicon* is found in people suffering from chilblains.

(iii)   The above climatic conditions can give rise to chilblains in both summer and winter, although we always tend to associate them with cold, damp winters.

TREATMENT

Treatment comes under the headings:–

(I) *PREVENTION* and (II) *CURE*.

(I) PREVENTION

(a)   Try to maintain a *'warm atmosphere'* around all parts of the body.

(b)   Wear *warm clothes* and cover areas of the body which we tend to expose to the weather. Wear gloves and stout footwear.

(c)   *Exercise* is good. The answer is not hugging a hot water-bottle or sitting near a fire.

(d)   *Plastic* or *rubber* shoes should not be warn indoors in cold weather.

(II) CURE
Consider two types of chilblain (a) *Broken* and (b) *Unbroken*. The treatment differs in each case.

(a) *BROKEN CHILBLAINS*
(i)   Bathe gently in warm water and apply a healing herbal ointment such as *Calendula* or *Comfrey*. Both of these preparations are obtainable from Herbal Stores.
(ii)   Paint *Garlic* juice on the broken area.

(b) *UNBROKEN CHILBLAINS*
Treatment is essentially under 3 headings.
(i)   *Improve* the *circulation* of the blood with a *stimulating tea* or *tisane*.
This treatment can apply also under the heading of 'Broken Chilblains'.
(ii)   Take a *Footbath* or *Handbath* before retiring.
(iii)   Treat the affected areas with *Compresses*.

(i)   *Improving the circulation of the blood*
Take *Angelica* 2 parts
        Lady's Mantle 2 parts
        Golden Rod 2 parts
        Hawthorn Flowers 2 parts
The preparation must be made each morning. Take 4 tablespoonsful of the mixed herbs and pour on 2 pints of boiling water. Allow the preparation to infuse for $\frac{1}{4}$ hour and a cupful can be taken 2 or 3 times a day.

(ii)   *The footbath or the handbath* should be taken regularly until the condition clears. The solution should be prepared as follows:–
Take *Vetch* 1 part
        Hawthorn 3 parts
        Shepherd's Purse 3 parts
        Sanicle 3 parts
To 5 tablespoonsful of the mixed herbs add 4 pints of boiling water. Allow this to stand for 10 minutes, strain and add cold water as required.

(iii)   *Treat the affected area with lukewarm compresses*
(a)   A good *compress* is make as follows:–
Take *Blessed Thistle* 2 parts
      Mallow Leaves 2 parts
      Sage 2 parts
      Coltsfoot Leaves 2 parts
Mix the herbs thoroughly and add 2 pints of boiling water to 3 tablespoonsful of the mixed herbs. Brew for 10 minutes, strain, and use the liquid to make a lukewarm compress.
(b)   Another *compress* could be made with the following herbs:–
Take *2 pinches* of each of these herbs, *Yarrow, Mullein, Marshmallow, Fir Shoots* and *Marigold.*
Add these to 2 pints of water, boil for 20 minutes, strain, and use the liquid for the *compress.*
(iv)   *Homely 'first-aid'* treatments can be tried.
(a)   Dip half a *Lemon* in *Salt* and gently rub on the chilblain.
(b)   Rub on a slice of *Onion.*
(c)   Paint on *Nettle Juice.*
(d)   Rub on the juice of freshly cut *House Leek,* as often as required.
(e)   A 'Romany Remedy' is to cut *raw potato* into slices and cover with salt. Allow to stand overnight, when it will turn black. Take a slice and rub it on unbroken skin. Allow it to dry. This gives instant relief. If applied frequently the chilblain quickly disappears.

DIET
To supply adequate amounts of calcium and silicon for the body's immediate needs these foods should be eaten:–
Cabbages (both raw and cooked), cheese, lettuce, spinach, milk, lemons and oranges, barley, figs, oats and strawberries, blackcurrant juice and lemon juice are also advised.

CONSULTANT OPINION
In treating chilblains the Consultant Herbalist might include the following herbs:–
(i)   *Capsicum* or *Cayenne* (Capsicum minimum). It has antiseptic properties, relieves the irritation and the itching and also improves the local circulation of blood.
(ii)   *Rhatany Root* (Krameria triandra) will reduce the swelling and heal the area.

(iii)   *Arnica* (Arnica montana) relieves the intense itching and irritation. It should *not* however, be used on broken chilblains, and it can produce dermatitis in some people.

Condition: COLDS

DEFINITION
The *common cold* called the 'scourge of every nation' is an infection of the lining membrane of the nose and its air passages.

CAUSES
It is a *virus* infection which predisposes to further invasion by *bacteria*. The spread is through coughing and sneezing. One cold does not give more than a few days' immunity and normally we have three to four colds a year, varying in intensity. Both sexes and all ages are involved.

IDENTIFICATION
There is a clear discharge from the nose which becomes thick and yellow after a day or two. This is at the time the bacteria invade. A slight sore throat is often the first sign of a cold and comes before the running nose. Headache is usual, sneezing is common and there is sometimes fever.
We say that the common cold is a week coming, and a week going, i.e. it usually lasts a fortnight from beginning to end, but if the cold is not adequately treated, then the complications of tonsillitis and bronchitis may follow.

TREATMENT
(a) PREVENTION
(i)   If you are not sure whether a cold is coming on, or perhaps something more serious such as flu, infuse 1oz of fresh or 1 teaspoonful of dried *Balm* with a pint of boiling water and take it very hot last thing at night, in wineglassful doses.
Don't hesitate but take it immediately the first symptoms arise.
(ii)   Make a tisane of *Feverfew* using 1 teaspoonful of dried leaves or

1oz green leaves. Infuse with a pint of boiling water. Take a wineglassful three times a day.

At the first signs of a sore throat, a tisane of *Self Heal* will ease the inflamed membranes.

(iii)   An infusion of 2 pinches of *Garden Thyme,* 2 pinches of *Wild Thyme,* to two pints of boiling water, and infused for 10 minutes, will prevent a lot of unpleasantness if taken as a course of 3-4 cupsful per day and starting at the beginning of winter.

(iv)   *Parsley* is rich in Vitamin C. Chop it up and eat it raw on any savoury dish or salad, or added to soup. It is a great preventative for colds.

(v)   The favourite Romany prescription to prevent a cold is to put *Elderberries* into an earthenware jar, cover with a lid and place in a slow oven. Leave until the juice begins to run then pour it off into a pan. Repeat this until all the juice has been extracted from the fruit, then squeeze the rest of the fruit through muslin.

To every 1 pint of juice add ½lb lump sugar, half a dozen *Cloves,* and a piece of bruised *Root Ginger*, bring to the boil, and simmer for 25-30 minutes. Strain into bottles, cork securely and drink diluted with hot water to taste.

(b) TO STOP A COLD IN EARLY STAGES

(i)   Make an infusion of *Basil*, 1 teaspoonful to 1 pint of boiling water. This will promote perspiration and drive out the cold.

or

(ii)   Pour boiling water over dry *Elderberry Flowers*, leave to infuse for a few minutes then add sugar. In addition to 'breaking up' a cold it will give a good night's sleep and calm the nerves.

TREATMENT – INHALATIONS

(i)   *Friars Balsam, Menthol* or *Eucalyptus* added to a jug of near boiling water, and the steam carrying the healing vapour, inhaled under a bath towel, may be comforting but not completely curative, especially if the sinuses and bronchial tubes are involved.

(ii)   Inhalations of *Olbas Oil* – for constitution see 'Catarrh'.

(iii)   Mix together 2 parts *Oregano* to 3 parts *Mint*, 3 parts *Thyme* and *May Flower Heads* 2 parts. Place 2 tablespoonsful of the mixture in 1 pint of boiling water. Inhale the vapour. Dry the face well and keep warm.

TREATMENT – TISANES

(i)   For a 'dry' cold, *Peppermint* tea or tisane will quickly relieve the symptoms. Use 1 teaspoonful of dried herb to 1 pint of boiling water and allow to 'brew'. Take 1 cupful as required.

(ii)   Fresh *orange* or *lemon juice* used in hot drinks will encourage perspiration to rid the body of its poisons.

(iii)   A tablespoonful of each of *Elderflowers*, *Peppermint*, and Yarrow, infused with 1 pint of boiling water, strained and take 1 large cupful going to bed (hot), and take the same 'brew' 3 times during the next day, and again on going to bed, and the cold will be quickly dispersed.

(iv)   Stew *Barberry Berries* with a little water, until they are soft, squeeze through a strainer pressing out all the juice with a wooden spoon. Add 3 pints of water to 1 pint of juice. This juice taken hot at night is guaranteed to induce perspiration to drive out a cold.

(v)   *Coltsfoot* tea sweetened with honey is an excellent remedy for colds. Use an infusion of the leaves. 1 teaspoonful of the dried leaves or 1oz of the fresh leaves to 1 pint of boiling water.

(vi)   A similar infusion of *Yarrow* will disperse a cold within 24 hours, leaving no trace of unpleasant catarrh or cough.

(vii)   A tea using *Thyme and Sage*. 1 teaspoonful of each to 1 pint of boiling water is excellent for the sore throat.

(viii) A gargle with *Sage Tisane* is popular for sore throats.

(ix)   We must remember that *Horseradish* will help to relieve the *catarrhal deafness* often associated with a cold. Take 1oz grated *Horseradish* root to 1 pint of boiling water. Let it stand for 15 minutes, strain and take 4 tablespoonsful twice a day. If the flavour is unacceptable mix in a little syrup of ginger or caraway.

DIET

Eat salads, radishes, horseradish, onions, turnips, leeks, figs and honey. In place of sweets take blackcurrant, grapefruit and lemon juice.

CONSULTANT OPINION

As one would expect the choice of Herbal therapies available to the Consultant for the treatment of the common cold are legion, but popular ones are:–
Hyssop (Hyssopus); *Yarrow* (Millefolium); *Elderberry* (Sambucus); *Sage* (Teucrium).

They are prescribed in medicinal doses using tinctures and liquid extracts of the herbs.

(i)   *Hyssop* (Hyssopus officinalis) is relaxing, promotes perspiration and helps to remove the offensive secretions from the nose, throat and bronchial tubes.

(ii)   *Yarrow* (Achillea millefolium) promotes sweating, reduces temperature, increases the flow of urine and reduces the swelling of the lining membrane of the passages affected.

(iii)   *Elder flowers* (Sambucus nigra) prevents catarrh and promotes sweating.

(iv)   *Wood Sage* (Teucrium scorodonia), prevents further infection of the area with other bacteria and reduces the swelling of the lining membranes of the passages. It has healing properties.

Condition: CIRCULATION

❀ ❀ ❀

DESCRIPTION

Circulation is described as the movement of blood through the various vessels of the body, to all parts of the body.

There are 3 kinds of circulation and each system has its own particular function. They are:–

(i)   The *Systemic or General* circulation in which purified blood, i.e. blood which has been reinforced with oxygen, and all impurities (toxins) have been removed, is pumped by the *heart* through the *arteries* of the body to the smaller *capillaries* in the superficial areas and extremities of the body.

On its way, this blood has accumulated the toxins of the body and has become deprived of its oxygen as it has passed through the various organs and working systems of the body. It returns to the heart as impure blood to be pumped to the *lungs,* and become the second circulation called:–

(ii)   The *Pulmonary circulation,* where the blood becomes recharged with oxygen and 'purified'.

(iii)   The third system is the *Portal Circulation* where blood is collected from behind the pancreas, and which is very rich in the products of digestion and conveyed to the *liver.* Here in the liver, the circulation breaks up into tiny capillaries. Blood leaves the liver by veins which enter the large veins going to the heart, to complete the circuit.

Circulation is maintained by the pumping action of the heart whose rhythm is controlled by a 'Pacemaker' situated in the heart muscle itself, and which consists of a group of special nerve cells which gives off electrical impulses.

DEFECTS

Defects in the *Circulation* are considered to be due to *three main groups* of causes:–

CAUSES

In the *first* group defective circulation may be the outcome of a heavily toxin-laden condition of the blood and blood vessels. This type is usually seen in heavily built people where it is felt that the external surface of the body is in a permanently 'half active' condition, resulting in a feeling of coldness and numbness in the extremities. The chief factors setting up this condition are usually faulty diet, and lack of exercise.

CAUSES

The *second group* showing a deficiency in their circulation can have a prolonged history of previous disease, suffer from nervous exhaustion, and exhibit excesses of all kinds, coupled with defective nutrition and poor assimulation by the body of the food that is eaten. They are excessively thin.

CAUSES

In the *third group* for various reasons the heart is unable to pump adequate blood through the system.

An *improved circulation* gives a feeling of warmth in the body.

TREATMENT

The treatment of *Poor Circulation* includes (i) *Baths* (ii) *Tisanes* (iii) *Culinary* uses in the kitchen.

(i)   *Lavender bath*. Pour 1 quart of boiling water over 4ozs blossoms. Let stand covered for $^1/_2$ hours. Strain the liquid and add it to the bath. Bathe for 10 minutes only 3 times a week. It has an invigorating and stimulating affect, and *should not be taken in the evening*.

(ii)   *Horsetail bath*
(a)   *Full bath.* Heat 5 tablespoonsful of dried chopped herb in 1 quart water. Boil for 1 minute. Stand for 20 minutes, strain and add to bath water at blood heat.
(b)   *Hand and foot bath.* Place 2-3 tablespoonsful dried herb in pint water, place the mixture in the bath water. Bathe hand or foot at moderate heat.
(iii)   *Rosemary bath.* Pour 1 quart boiling water over 2 handfuls of leaves. Let it stand covered for 20 minutes. Strain the liquid and add to the bath water. Bathe at body temperature for 10 minutes, 3 times a week. *Rest at least ½ hour after the bath. Do not bathe in the evening.*
(iv)   *Scotch Pine Bath.* Place 4ozs pine needles in 1 pint of water. Boil for 1 minute. Let it stand for 20 minutes. Add to the bath water and bathe at body temperature for 10 minutes.
(v)   *Mustard foot bath.* Use 1 teaspoonful of *Mustard* powder to a foot bath of hot water tisane is helpful.
(i)   *Hawthorn Tea.* Take 2 teaspoonsful of the leaves or blossoms, or equal parts of both. Add 1 cup of boiling water. Stand for 20 minutes and take 1 cupful as a hot drink, sweetened with honey 2-3 times daily for several weeks or months.
(ii)   Infuse a *pinch* each of the following herbs:–
Aniseed, Mint, Sage, Basil and *Vervain* with 1 cup of boiling water. Take a cup of the tisane regularly.
The following herbs in regular use in the *kitchen*, and which improve circulation include:– *Garlic, Ginger, Mustard, Black Pepper, Cayenne Pepper, Sage* and *Basil*.

CONSULTANT OPINION
Popular with the Herbal Consultants are
(i)   *Prickly Ash Bark* (Zanthoxylum americanum). Which improves circulatory insufficiency in the extremities and is usually combined with *Bayberry Bark* and *Ginger*.
(ii)   *Hawthorn* (Crataegus oxyacantha). It is used combined with *night-blooming cereus* in the treatment of disorderly circulation related to heart conditions.
(iii)   *Maiden Hair Tree* (Ginkgo biloba). Is used for arterial circulation failure in the extremities. It is prepared from fresh leaves commercially and taken as a medicine.

Condition: PAIN IN THE STOMACH: COLIC

DEFINITION

Nature's danger signal. Never ignore it. It is foolhardy to be brave about *abdominal pain,* which although often due to trivia like dietary indiscretion, constipation, or mild food-poisoning, can point to a more *serious* condition, especially if the pain is severe and recent, if the abdomen is distended or hard and very tender to pressure, if there is nausea vomiting, or if there is blood or tarry colour in the motions.

Severe abdominal pain lasting several hours after previous good health requires IMMEDIATE INVESTIGATION BY A DOCTOR, AND THE SOONER, THE SAFER.

Never take a *purgative* when suffering from unexplained abdominal pain, even if the bowels are constipated.

With a *true colic* the pains are very sharp, and agonising bouts cause writhing and doubling up, and sometimes they are associated with a cold feeling and vomiting.

The abdomen is not hard during the pain spasms, nor is it distended.

Pressing the abdomen in a case of *true colic* slightly relieves the pain, but not so of any other abdominal condition.

In colic, which is usually understood to be *intestinal colic,* the pain is usually gripping in the upper abdomen, and around the navel, there are gurgling sounds and patches of gas, and sometimes vomiting.

CAUSES

(i)   *Infection* which we call *Enteritis.*
(ii)   *Irritation* from indigestible or tainted foods.
(iii)   The *toxins,* i.e. poisons from some fevers.
(iv)   *Constipation.*

TREATMENT

(i)   *Chamomile Tea* is one of the best first aid remedies. Using about 6 heads of flowers to 1 pint of boiling water and infusing. It soothes the nerves and strengthens the digestion.

(ii)   *Peppermint Tea* and honey is a very suitable drink. Add a teaspoonful of aniseed. The dose is a teaspoonful frequently.

(iii) *Thyme Tea* is also a very valuable drink in this condition.

(iv) A hot infusion of the following ingredients:– 2 pinches of *Lavender,* 2 pinches of *Lime Flowers,* 2 pinches of *Marjoram* and 2 pinches of *Mallow.* Use 2 pints of boiling water and take 2 cupsful per day.

(v) Local heat in the form of a *Linseed Poultice* or just an ordinary hot water-bottle is very comforting.

(vi) A tisane using 4 herbs consists of *Juniper Berries, Camomile flowers, Wormwood,* and *Yarrow.* Mix in equal parts. Infuse 1 teaspoonful in ½ cup of boiling water. Take ½ cup unsweetened.

(vii) For *Colic in infants* use 4 parts *Fennel Seed* to 3 parts *Water Mint* leaves, 2 parts *Camomile Flowers,* and 1 part *Fragrant Valerian.* Add ½ teaspoonful of the mixture to 1½ cups of boiling water for 5 minutes, then strain. Give 5 or 6 doses during the day in warm milk or by itself. Dose is one teaspoonful.

CONSULTANT OPINION

For an uncomplicated intestinal colic a Consultant Herbalist may make use of tincture or liquid extracts of one or more herbs of this popular list:– (i) *Acorus;* (ii) *Alpinia;* (iii) *Carum;* (iv) *Cinnamonum Cassia;* (v) *Dioscorea;* (vi) *Nepeta Cataria;* (vii) *Petroselinum;* (viii) *Zingiber.*

(i) *Calamus Root* (Acorus Calamus). Eases gripping pains, and expels flatulence, reduces the spasms and cramps of colic, and promotes perspiration.

(ii) *Colic Root* (Alpinia officinarum). Eases gripping pains and promotes sweating.

(iii) *Caraway* (Carum carvi). Expels flatulence, reduces the cramps of colic and prevents infection with germs.

(iv) *Chinese Cinnamon* (Cinnamonium cassia). Prevents infection with germs, prevents vomiting and diarrhoea, reduces stomach cramps, and expels flatulence.

(v) *Wild Yam Root* (Dioscorea villosa). Reduces inflammation and stomach cramps.

(vi) *Catmint* (Nepeta cataria). Reduces fever, calms the nervous system, reduces stomach cramps and prevents diarrhoea. It expels flatulence also.

(vii) *Parsley Root* (Petroselinum crispum). Reduces cramps and expels flatulence. It also inhibits the multiplication of germs in the intestine.

(viii) *Ginger* (Zingiber officinale). Expels flatulence, reduces stomach cramps and promotes sweating.

Condition: CONSTIPATION

DEFINITION
Constipation is undue delay in the passage of the residue of a meal. Concern has been registered over the bowels since the time of the ancient Egyptians who used *enemas* to rid the bowel of this waste and indeed in the medieval herbal books over 50 per cent of the 'concoctions' were *purges*.

IDENTIFICATION
There are prolonged gaps between evacuations or motions and difficulty in passing them.
We must remember however, that there is no law about the bowels being opened once a day. Each person has an individual pattern, and having a motion once, twice or every other day can still be healthy.
With *constipation* which, as described above is the undue 'delay' in the individual, there is usually a feeling of *uneasiness* or *discomfort* in the abdomen.
Headaches, furred tongue and wind are not the usual accompaniment of constipation itself, but are caused by the treatments we tend to take to 'dose ourselves', i.e. aperients or laxatives. Women tend to be 'sufferers' from constipation more than men.

CAUSES
(i)   *Faulty habits* from childhood, ignoring or resisting the feeling of wanting to pass a motion because of laziness, inconvenience, or 'lack of time'. The feeling passes off, and the bowels' warning being ignored, also passes off.
(ii)   *Chemical laxatives and purgatives* act to produce a motion by irritating the bowels and this is how they work. The food is rushed along the digestive tract so quickly that it arrives in the 'evacuation part' of the intestine in an undigested state. Here it decomposes, and gives off offensive gases. If unknowingly we consider this to be due to

constipation, the temptation persists to repeat the dose of purgative. This makes matters worse, giving rise to those well-known feelings of malaise, headache, furred tongue and wind. Distension develops. In this condition bad dreams can occur.

(iii)   *Weak muscles* as in old age, after pregnancy, and in people who are unable to exercise sufficiently, and lead a sedentary life.

(iv)   *A spasm of the bowel* known as spastic constipation. This condition is caused by stress or anxiety and whilst the spasm lasts the motion cannot pass.

(v)   A local *painful condition* such as piles can disturb the 'habit' of the person.

(vi)   *Inadequate and unsuitable diet* either in amount, or fluid, or in roughage. The stimulus of the 'waste' is not enough for a call to have a motion.

(vii)   *Strange surroundings,* e.g. an unfamiliar lavatory seat as on holiday, is sufficient to disturb the reflexes which start off the wish to go to the toilet.

(viii) *Constipation alternating with diarrhoea* is a danger signal of something more serious and your doctor should be consulted.

TREATMENT

Let us consider *PREVENTION* first:–

(i)   Try not to break the natural 'habit' which the body has acquired – set aside an adequate period of time for the 'job', and *never* fail to respond to the urge to have a motion.

(ii)   *Exercise* well. Particularly if you are older. Exercise tones up the muscles and gives a better mental outlook. Swimming is an excellent exercise.

FOR ADULTS IN DELICATE HEALTH

Make up the following tisane. Take *Alder Buckthorn Bark* 4 parts, *Ash Leaves* 2 parts, *Alder Flowers* 2 parts, *Mint* 2 parts. Add 2 teaspoonsful of this mixture to a cup of boiling water. Strain, drink 1 or 2 cups of the tisane on retiring to bed at night.

FOR ADULTS IN GOOD HEALTH

Take *Senna Leaves* 3 parts, *Mint Leaves* 3 parts, *Chamomile Flowers* 1 part, *Marjoram* 3 parts. Use 2 teaspoonsful of the mixture to a cup of boiling water, strain, drink 1 or 2 cups of the tisane on retiring to bed at night.

FOR PROLONGED TREATMENT IN CHRONIC CASES SUCH AS SLIMMING
Take *Alder Buckthorn Bark* 4 parts, *Baldo Leaves* 2 parts, *Blackthorn Flowers* 2 parts, *Heartsease* 2 parts. Take 2 teaspoonsful of the mixture to 1 cup of boiling water, strain, drink 1 or 2 cups in the evening on retiring to bed.
Eat sensibly and avoid getting cold.
There are several popular everyday 'cures' for constipation. They include:–

(i)   1 teaspoonful of honey taken in a cup of hot water before breakfast. Use 1 teaspoonful per cup and take as hot as possible.

(ii)   *Dandelion* coffee should replace ordinary coffee.

(iii)   *Slippery elm* mixed with equal parts of warm water and honey used before breakfast and before going to bed at night is a curable agent.

(iv)   *Elder bark* powdered and drunk in warm water is a good laxative.

(v)   *Icelandic moss* can be lightly boiled and the water kept to cure constipation.

(vi)   *Rhubarb* sweetened with honey, or black molasses is one of the best treatments for constipation sufferers.

(vii)   *Apricots* mashed with a little honey are very beneficial.

(viii) An infusion of a pinch of *Aniseed*, a pinch of *Chamomile*, a pinch of *Vervain* and a pinch of *Basil* to a cup of boiling water is very acceptable. 1 or 2 cups per day will cure.

DIET
Plenty of fruit and fluid is advised, but do not make a fetish of having one particular thing, say prunes for breakfast, include these in your diet:– apples, apricots, bran, beetroot, cucumbers, currants, celery, lettuce, oranges, prunes, strawberries, tomatoes. Watercress or parsley, eaten daily is a certain cure. Liquorice is the only sweet to be allowed to constipated patients.

CONSULTANT OPINION
A very wide choice of herbs is available to the Consultant Herbalist for the treatment of constipation. A popular choice would be the use of:–
(i) *Cassia fruit;* (ii) *Cassia leaf;* (iii) *Juglans;* (iv) *Rhamnus;* (v) *Veronicastrom.*
(i) and (ii) *Cassia fruit* (Senna pods) and *Cassia leaf* (Senna leaf).

There are both *Alexandrian senna* and *Tinnevelly senna* available. The leaf is stronger than the fruits – senna is a strong purgative.

(iii)   *Butternut bark* (Juglans cinerea) has a milder reaction than the senna, and is used in chronic constipation with dyspepsia.

(iv)   *Cascara* (Rhamnus purshiana) is a mild purgative.

(v)   *Black root* (Veronicastrum virginicum) is a mild purgative and is used chiefly for a chronic constipation associated with faulty liver function.

Condition: CORNS

❀ ❀ ❀

DEFINITION

Corns are a local excessive production of a horny material in the skin called keratin.

CAUSES

They are caused by pressure on the skin and frequently occur on the feet as a result of wearing ill-fitting footwear.

TREATMENT

(i)   Corns should be treated with equal portions of *soft soap* and *roasted onions* mixed up and used as a poultice.

(ii)   Apply a clove of crushed *garlic* to the corn and protect the surrounding skin with sticking-plaster.

(iii)   Corns can be eliminated with a plaster of *ivy leaves* and *celandine leaves* soaked in *vinegar* and changed frequently.

(iv)   *Dandelion Juice* put fresh on to the corn every night has been found very effective.

(v)   *Lemon Juice* placed neat on the corn night and morning has produced very satisfactory results.

(vi)   *Celandine Juice* is a time-honoured remedy.

(vii)   If a *Swede Turnip* is hollowed out and filled with salt and allowed to stay for 24 hours. The corn can be bathed with the liquid night and morning.

Condition: CRAMP

❀ ❀ ❀

DEFINITION
Cramp is a sudden continuous spasm or contraction of muscles. It is very painful.

CAUSES
It is caused by a serious imbalance of mineral salts in the diet, particularly magnesium, calcium and silicon.

TREATMENT
(i)   Massage *Clove Oil* diluted with *Olive Oil* into the affected area.
(ii)   *Tincture of Myrrh* can also be massaged into the affected muscles.
(iii)   *Catmint leaves* can be crushed and massaged on to the muscles.
(iv)   Sir Frances Bacon in his time, recommended that *Periwinkle* (Vinca major) is a good remedy for cramp and prescribed bands of the green stems to be tied around the limbs.
Tisanes are well accepted for this condition.
(i)   Take equal parts of *Silverweed, Balm leaves and Chamomile flowers*. Infuse 1 teaspoonful in ½ cup of boiling water. Sweeten with honey and take 1-1½ cups a day in mouthful doses.
(ii)   The Romanies have an excellent cramp cure.
Take 1oz each of *Vervain, Prickly Ash Bark,* and *Black Cohosh root*. This amount will make 3 brewings which will cure the condition. Boil ⅓ of these mixed herbs in a pint of water for 20 minutes, cool, strain, and add 1 tablespoonful of 'Composition Essence'. (The herbs and the essence can be obtained from the Herb Shop.) Take a wineglassful of the brew between meals.
Footbaths and handbaths will help to relieve cramps since they are comforting and relaxing. Take a handful of *Yarrow,* a crushed head of *Garlic,* half a handful of *Chamomile,* half a handful of *Celandine,* a handful of *Sage* and a handful of *Thyme,* to 2 pints of water, leave the herbs in the bath as it is being used. Repeat the treatment if this is necessary.

DIET

Take black molasses and the following foods rich in the essential minerals to ease and cure this condition.

Raw cabbage, cheese, lemons, lettuce, milk, oranges and spinach. Barley, figs, oats and strawberries are particularly rich in the mineral silicon. Blackberries, raspberries and carrots are favoured by the Romanies.

CONSULTANT OPINION

The popular herbs used by the Consultant Herbalist include:–

(i)   *Guelder Rose* (Viburnun opulus). Reduces spasm and calming the nerves concerned.

(ii)   *Colic Root* (Dioscorea villosa). Is anti-inflammatory, reduces spasm and promotes mild perspiration.

(iii)   *Prickly Ash Bark; Prickly Ash Berries* (Zanthoxylum americanum). Stimulates the circulation, relieving the spasm, and promotes mild perspiration.

(iv)   *Valerian Root* (Valeriana officinalis). Reduces spasm of muscles, eases pain and calms the activity of the nerves concerned.

Condition: CYSTITIS

❀ ❀ ❀

DEFINITION

Cystitis is the name given to inflammation of the urinary bladder. It can affect any age, and women are more prone to suffer from it than men.

CAUSES

Predisposing causes of cystitis include, a chill, constipation, over-indulgence in alcohol, and incomplete emptying of the bladder when passing urine. The actual causes of cystitis are numerous, but the most prevelant one, is invasion of the lining of the bladder with the germs of infection, i.e. micro-organisms.

IDENTIFICATION

Pain is felt in the lower part of the abdomen and between the legs. There is a desire to pass water, even just after the bladder has been emptied. Stronger pain may be felt in the area at the end of the act of passing urine. The urine may feel 'scalding' as it is passed, blood may be passed and the urine itself may become thick and ropey.

Fever is not always present, and the sufferer may not always feel ill. The condition may be persistent, with the symptoms less severe, if the condition is not treated as urgent.

TREATMENT

If the condition does not show any signs of subsiding after an initial course of treatment, one must *CONSULT A DOCTOR*, as investigations beyond the scope of the Consultant Herbalist must be undertaken to determine the exact cause of the condition, and specific treatment initiated for any condition which may be producing cystitis as a secondary effect.

It is imperative that throughout treatment ample quantities of *bland fluids,* e.g. lemon barley should be taken.

Several very effective tisanes can be prepared for the treatment of cystitis. Popular ones are included in the following instructions.

(i)   1oz of the dried roots of *Couch grass* boiled for 5 minutes in 1½ pints of water. Strain and take a wineglassful 5 or 6 times a day.

(ii)   *Buchu tea* using 1oz to 1 pint of boiling water, straining and taking a wineglassful as required.

(iii)   *Parsley Piert* tea made in the same manner and taken as the buchu tea.

(iv)   Using more than 1 herb, which is common practice with the Consultant Herbalist make up:–

1 part *Lovage root,* 1 part *Parsley seed,* 3 parts *Barberry leaves.* Of this mixture of herbs use 1½ teaspoonsful to a cupful of water, bring to the boil quickly, strain and take ½ cupful of the mixture 3 times a day.

(v)   A valuable recipe is as follows:–

1oz *Burdock seed,* 1oz *Dandelion,* 1oz *Marshmallow Root,* 1oz *Tansy,* 1oz *Uva Ursi* (bearberry). Mix the herbs well and put them into 2 quarts of boiling water. Simmer until the quantity of liquid is reduced by one half. When cool take a wineglassful every 2 hours the first day, and every 3 hours on succeeding days until the condition has cleared.

(vi)   A popular Romany recipe is to take a handful of *Nettles* and a handful of *Tansy,* put them into a quart of boiling water, brew for 10 minutes, strain and drink when the liquid is cool – a cupful at a time.

(vii) *St. John's Wort* tea has been in use for a considerable time. Using 1oz of the herb or 1 teaspoonful of the dried herb to 1 pint of boiling water. Infuse for 10 minutes, and take ½ teacupful 3 or 4 times a day.

DIET

Sugar and sweets must be avoided. Since constipation *must* be avoided, fruits and salads are an essential part of the daily diet. Watercress, parsley, celery and likewise carrots are valuable articles of food to be included. Lemon and orange juice should be freely available.

CONSULTANT OPINION

As previously mentioned a trained Herbalist knows how to make up herbal prescriptions, including several valuable herbs, to be taken according to instructions given.

The choice may include:– (i) *Agathosma;* (ii) *Agropyron;* (iii) *Arctostaphylos;* (iv) *Eryngium;* (v) *Hydrangea;* (vi) *Parietoria;* (vii) *Piper methysticum;* (viii) *Zea Mays.*

(i)   *Buchu leaves* (Agathosma betulina) which is a urinary antiseptic and encourages discharge of the urine.

(ii)   *Couch grass* (Agropyron repens) increases the discharge of the urine to wash away the infection.

(iii)   *Bearberry leaves (Uva-Ursi)* (Arctostophylos Uva-Ursi) is a urinary antiseptic, reduces the swelling of the lining membrane of the bladder, and encourages the discharge of urine.

(iv)   *Sea Holly* (Eryngium maritinum) promotes the flow of urine.

(v)   *Seven barks* (Hydrangea arborescens) increases the flow of urine to rid the bladder of gravel and infection.

(vi)   *Pellitory-of-the wall* (Parietaria diffusa) both soothes and protects the inflammed lining of the bladder and promotes the flow of urine.

(vii)   *Kava* (Piper methysticum) prevents the invasion of the area with bacteria, takes away the pain of spasm, and calms the irritation of the bladder. It also promotes the flow of urine.

(viii)   *Corn Silk* (Zea Mays) promotes the flow of urine.

Condition: DEBILITY

❈ ❈ ❈

DEFINITION
Debility denotes general body weakness or loss of power and vitality. It is often a sign of anaemia.

CAUSES
Considered to be due to a deficiency of essential mineral salts and vitamins in the body.

SIGNS AND SYMPTOMS
(i)   There is a general feeling of being 'below the weather'.
(ii)   Life has lost its zest.
(iii)   Transient giddiness may be present.

TREATMENT
(a)   A *tonic to the whole system* in the treatment of General Debility, and one favoured by the Romanies is *Centaury Tea* or *Tisane*. Use 1 teaspoonful of the dried herb and to it add 1 pint of boiling water. Infuse (brew) for 10 minutes, then take a wineglassful dose or 4 tablespoonsful every 4 hours.
(b)   *To improve the body's vitality.* Use a 'compound' tisane. Take equal parts of *Balm* and *St. John's Wort*. Mix the herbs together well. Take 1 teaspoonful of the mixture and to them add 1 pint of boiling water. Infuse for 10 minutes then take 1-1½ cupsful over a whole day, sweetened with honey and in mouthful doses. This should be taken over an extended period.

DIET
Is very important:−
(i)   Take *Black Molasses* daily and twice a day.
(ii)   *Honey* should be used instead of sugar.
(iii)   Increase the *protein*, i.e. body-building material in the diet, take red meats, chicken, fish, eggs, cheese.
(iv)   The diet should include *fresh green salads* and fruit.
(v)   *Home-made lemonade,* made with fresh *Lemons* and sweetened with honey, and flavoured with a pinch of *Nutmeg* or *Cinnamon*, is highly advisable.

CONSULTANT OPINION

General *tonics,* favoured and used by Consultant Herbalists include:–

(i)   *Lucerne* (Medicago sativa). It is nutrient, a source of the vitamins A, C and E and of the mineral salts calcium, potassium, phosphorus and iron.

(ii)   *Fenugreek Seeds* (Trigonella foenum-graecum). They are nutritive and stimulate the appetite.

(iii)   *Peruvian Bark* (Chinchona succirubra) has a bitter taste. It stimulates and increases the appetite.

Condition: DIABETES MELLITUS (SUGAR DIABETES)

❀ ❀ ❀

DEFINITION

Diabetes mellitus or *Sugar Diabetes* as it is commonly called, is a body dysfunction which produces sugar in the urine, excess sugar in the blood and a disturbance in the way the body utilises fats and proteins.

DESCRIPTION

Consider the body to be a machine or engine which science has proved it to be. An engine burns coal to produce heat and energy, and man burns similar fuel in a similar way, the fuel being the food he eats. His chief fuel is the carbon contained in sugar and starchy foods which together are called *carbohydrates.* Starchy foods such as flour, bread and potatoes become sugar when digested and behave exactly like sugar itself, in the body.

The *diabetic* unfortunately cannot use and burn sugar and starch properly, and his illness arises from this. When such foods are eaten, sugar is not burned normally, but accumulates in the body, it overflows and is wasted in the urine, making the patient weak, poisoning him, and producing the symptoms of illness. Other kinds of food which the body uses as fuel besides the carbohydrates are the albuminous foods of animal origin, such as meat, fish and eggs (known as *proteins*), and the *fats.* These also produce sugar indirectly in the body, and when sugar is not being burned properly in the diabetic, protein and fat also cannot be completely burned and, give rise to poisonous acids (acetone bodies) which affect the health unfavourably.

These dangerous acids accumulate when too much protein and fat are eaten, and for this reason *it is not safe to treat diabetes merely by restricting the starch and sugar in the diet.*

When a normal person eats sugar or starchy foods, a gland behind the stomach called the pancreas produces a substance called *INSULIN* which uses the sugar properly. To start combustion a fire requires a match – *insulin* provides this in the human body, and the pancreas provides exactly the right amount to deal correctly with the amount of carbohydrate eaten. In *diabetes* the pancreas is diseased and cannot produce enough insulin to deal with the sugar. A *mild case* can still produce some insulin, a *severe* case very little, if any.

PREDISPOSING CAUSES

There are many predisposing causes to this condition. They include:–
(i) *Age.* Diabetes can occur at all ages, but less commonly at the extreme of life. (ii) *Sex.* Females predominate. (iii) *Heredity.* There is a tendency for the condition to be present within the family. (iv) *Race.* Jews are prone to diabetes. (v) *Habits.* Over-eating and lack of exercise. (vi) *Nervous Shock.*

SIGNS AND SYMPTOMS

The onset of the disease may be gradual or sudden, the patient complaining of thirst, a large appetite and increasing weakness. In some cases there is a loss of weight, often marked in young subjects. Complications of the conditions include:–

(i)   *Skin lesions* – Boils, carbuncles, itching of the skin (pruritus) especially around the anus, vulva and on the penis.

(ii)   *Hardening of the Arteries* and *Increased Blood Pressure* with gangrene of the toes in elderly patients.

(iii)   *Diseases of the Kidneys* with albumen in the urine.

(iv)   *Eye changes* – they may include cataract (opacity of the lens) and small haemorrhages.

(v)   Involvement of the *Nervous System* especially in the lower limbs, producing tingling, pain, and loss of reflex action.

The *daily quantity of urine* is increased, it is pale in colour and sugar can be detected clinically by means of a simple test using a 'strip' which, when moistened with urine turns blue if sugar is present. This test is known as the clinistix test.

The most severe complication of diabetes is *Diabetic Coma* where the patient can become unconscious. There are 2 kinds.

(i)   *Hyperglycaemic Coma* when one of the products of disordered metabolism (ketones) collect in the body.

(ii)   *Hypoglycaemic Coma* occurring when either too much insulin or too little food have been taken.

TREATMENT

The first step in treatment is to try *diet,* and best results are obtained by eating a 'balanced' diet containing the same amount of carbohydrate and of protein and fat, every day. By using what is known as the *'line Ration' Diet Scheme,* a correct diet can easily be arranged and the patient learns to vary his food to suit his appetite and his income.

Any Consultant Herbalist or any Orthodox Practitioner has the use of this *Line Diet* issued as a card, and a certain number of rations are prescribed for one day. One *ration* is one complete line, and consists of one *black* and one *red* portion. Any black portion can be added to any red portion to make one ration, but two black portions or two red portions must *not* be combined to make a ration. The *black* portions are the foods containing carbohydrates. The *red* portions are the foods containing protein and fats.

It is for your Consultant to advise the *numbers of blacks and reds* to be taken, and to issue you with the *Line Ration Diet.*

Scheme Card

If you are taking *Insulin,* the correct balance between your diet and insulin must always be maintained. *NEVER STOP TAKING INSULIN WITHOUT YOUR CONSULTANT'S ORDERS.*

HERBAL TREATMENTS

A herb has been discovered in Argentina which is said to cure this illness even in advanced stages. It is PHYLLANTHUS SELLOWIANUS, but it is not easy to acquire.

There are 3 different herbal teas which have been tried and found to be helpful. This one has been used for many generations:–

1oz *Agrimony,* 1oz *Clivers,* 1oz *Dandelion Root,* 1oz *Juniper Berries,* 1oz *Parsley Piert* should be mixed together and placed in half a gallon of boiling water. This is simmered until only 1 quart remains. A wineglassful is drunk every 2 hours.

The second involves the use of the following herbs:– *Dandelion, Golden Seal, Lady's Mantle, Meadowsweet, Queen of the Meadow* and

Bistort Flowers and leaves (used either individually or mixed), and using 1oz of the fresh herb or ½ teaspoonful of powdered herb to 1 pint of boiling water. The dose is a wineglassful 3 times a day.

The third, long recommended is to take 2oz *Agrimony*, 2oz *Bistort Root*, 2oz *Meadow Fern Berries*, 2oz *Prickly Ash Berries*. The herbs are mixed and put into ½ gallon of boiling water simmered down to 1 quart. ¼oz *Cayenne Pepper* is thrown in before removing from the heat. The dose is one wineglassful every 3 hours.

The Romanies recommend boiling 1oz of the herb *Periwinkle* in 1½ pints of water for 10 minutes and taking a wineglassful 3 times a day.

Dietetic and *Herbal Treatment* by a *qualified person* are indicated. *DO NOT ATTEMPT TO TREAT THE CONDITION WITHOUT ADVICE.*

All cases of Diabetes are *individual*, and none of the herbal substances recommended here will necessarily prove infallible for any individual patient.

CONSULTANT OPINION

The Consultant Herbalist may find assistance in using the following herbs:–

(i)   *Goat's Rue* (Galega officinalis). It reduces the level of sugar in the blood.

The response is gradual over a period of time. If the patient is on insulin therapy it can remain so. The therapeutic dose is adjusted according to the concentration of sugar in both the blood and the urine.

(ii)   *Sweet Sumach* (Rhus aromatica) is reputed to lower the concentration of sugar in the blood.

(iii)   *Jambul* (Syzygium cumini), is also reputed to have similar qualities as above.

(iv)   *Nettle* (Urtica dioica) has similar properties to Sweet Sumach and Jambul, as far as lowering the sugar content of the blood is concerned.

Condition: DIARRHOEA

❀ ❀ ❀

DEFINITION

Diarrhoea means passing frequent stools or motions, which are loose and watery and more frequently than the individual's normal bowel habit. It is an exhausting condition which often robs the body of much needed mineral salts and vitamins. If there is a frequent desire to pass a motion without its consistency being abnormal, we do not call this diarrhoea.

TYPES OF DIARRHOEA
The motions passed in diarrhoea can vary considerably:–

(i)   Yellow in colour, resembling pea or lentil soup and containing undigested food which has been hurried along by the bowel without giving time for digestion.

(ii)   Bulky and greasy, but without pain. This means that there has been a failure to digest fats in the food.

(iii)   There can be much pain when the motion is passed. This will always be the case when blood and mucus (slime) are passed.

(iv)   If diarrhoea alternates with constipation it should always be considered as a danger sign to the beginning of more serious bowel ailment.

Diarrhoea can be described as either ACUTE or CHRONIC, by *ACUTE* we mean rapid and severe whilst *CHRONIC* means that it is a lengthy condition, and the reverse of ACUTE.

CAUSES OF ACUTE DIARRHOEA
Included under this heading are:– (i) *Virus gastro-enteritis;* (ii) *Food Poisoning;* (iii) *Bacillary Dysentery;* (iv) *Traveller's Diarrhoea;* (v) *Too much fruit;* (vi) *Typhoid Fever* and (vi) *Part of other acute illnesses such as infective hepatitis.*

CAUSES OF CHRONIC DIARRHOEA
Here are included (i) *Inflammation of the large bowel or colon,* called *COLITIS;* (ii) *Poor absorption* of the products of digestion. The motion is offensive and porridgy and there is flatulence (wind) and (iii) *Functional or Nervous Diarrhoea,* set off by eating unusual food or by emotional upset.

TREATMENT
If Diarrhoea is accompanied by a fever, i.e. a rise in body temperature the doctor must *always* be consulted.

(i)   A very old remedy for all acute diarrhoea and called *Dr. Slack's*

Cholera Syrup has been in use since the end of the last century. It reads:– Take a good handful of *Blackberry Roots*, put them into a pan with two teaspoonsful each of *Ground Nutmeg*, *Cloves* and *Cinnamon*. Pour on a quart of cold water, boil slowly for 20 minutes, strain, add 1¹/₂lbs of lump sugar and simmer again until a scum rises. Clear this off with a spoon and allow the herbs to cool. Then add 4ozs *Brandy*, bottle it, and keep it in a cool place.

The dose for a *child* is 1 teaspoonful every time the bowels are opened; for a *youth* is 1 tablespoonful, again every time the bowels are moved, and the adult is advised to take a wineglassful under the same conditions.

(ii)   Two teaspoonfuls of *Composition Essence* can be taken in 2 tablespoonfuls of cold milk, three times a day or more frequently. *Composition Essence* contains *Ginger, Cayenne, Cardamoms, Cinnamon* and *Bayberry* and the essence already prepared is readily available at any Herb or Health Store.

(iii)   *Arrowroot Powder* – already prepared and purchased from any health shop. My parents would buy it from the corner grocer's shop in my early years! The *Arrowroot Powder* is mixed with warm milk to a thin paste, and a dose of 1-3 dessertspoonsful of the mixture might suffice. This could be repeated if necessary after 4 hours.

Arrowroot powder can be taken alone from a spoon. It is unpleasant, but speedily effective.

(iv)   *Slippery Elm Root* (unmalted) and bought from any good chemist or health store is very popular. Made according to instructions into a gruel with water or milk, and taken three times a day. It is very soothing.

(v)   Equal parts of *Raspberry Leaf* and *Agrimony,* either the leaves or flowers, and take as follows, will arrest diarrhoea. Infuse 1oz to 1 pint. Wineglassful doses can be taken three times a day, either warm or cold, or *Agrimony Tea* alone can be taken. Use 1oz *Agrimony* to 1 pint of water, simmer gently for 15 minutes keeping the lid on the pot. It can be sweetened with brown sugar and a wineglassful dose taken before meals.

(vi)   If *colic* is really bad with indigestion, make an infusion of *Spearmint,* strain, and when cold sweeten with honey and add 1 teaspoonful of *Essence of Aniseed* to the pint. Dose:– 1 teaspoonful frequently.

(vii)   The Pharmaceutical Co. Cupal markets a *Diarrhoea Suspension* for 'the treatment' of mild diarrhoea of short duration. It contains a kaolin mixture which removes the poisons from the bowels, whilst the herbs cinnamon, nutmeg and clove oils disperse and expel the flatulence and remove the cramps. It is manufactured under the name 'KAO-C' and suspensions suitable for both children and adults are available.

(viii) *Blackberries* can be eaten freely.

(ix)   *Nettle Juice* can be taken neat or in cold water.

(x)   *Mint Sprigs* can be chewed fresh from the garden.

(xi)   A good *preventative* for diarrhoea and mild enough for children to take is *Meadowsweet tea*. Make tea with the flowers, strain and allow to cool before taking it.

DIET

Do not take anything *hot,* and refrain from eating any *meat*.

Take:– *Boiled fish,* with very little butter, on a small helping of bread or toast. *Water Biscuits* and small amounts of *dry, hard cheese* are tolerated by the body. So are *rice, sago* and *tapioca puddings*. No greens, however, should be taken, likewise very little *potato*.

As progress is maintained, lightly boiled or poached *eggs* can be introduced and a small helping of *cooked greens* and *potatoes*.

Macaroni, semolina and *milk puddings* with simple *sponge cake* and *custard* are accepted, likewise *fruit jellies* such as *blackcurrant* and also baked *apple*. *Tripe* can be introduced, and marmite on toast is allowed.

CONSULTANT OPINION

Consultant Herbalists have a very wide and varied choice of herbs in the treatment of diarrhoea. Here are some of them:–

(i)   *Greater Burnet* (Sanguisorba officinalis) is popular in the treatment of *acute* diarrhoea. It is astringent, i.e. it is binding, causing contraction of the tissues to be treated, and it also tends to control bleeding.

(ii)   *Oak Bark* (Quercus robur) is an astringent, used in acute diarrhoea and is taken in frequent small doses.

(iii)   *Germander* (Teucrium chamaedrys) inhibits the growth of the organisms which cause trouble. It prevents inflammation, and is specially indicated in the treatment of summer diarrhoea in infants.

(iv)   *Wild Yam Root or Colic Root* (Dioscorea villosa) reduces the inflammation, helps to remove the colic and promotes mild sweating.

(v)   *Sweet Flag or Calamus* (Acorus calamus). The root is used. It removes colic, expels the flatulence and promotes sweating to rid the body of its poisons.

(vi)   *Black Catechu* (Acacia catechu) is both antiseptic and astringent, and is used in the treatment of chronic diarrhoea, often in combination with agrimony and oak bark.

(vii)   *American Cranesbill* (Geranium maculatum) is used for the treatment of diarrhoea particularly in the young and the old. It is astringent, and controls bleeding.

(viii) *Jambul* (Syzygium cumini) is a herb from India and the East Indies. In practice it is often combined with oak bark, raspberry leaves and sweet flag. It is very popular in the treatment of diarrhoea with griping pains.

Lastly:–

(ix)   *Hemlock Spruce* (Tsuga canadensis) comes from North America. It is astringent, controls bowel infections, and promotes sweating. It is often used in combination with oak bark and black catechu.

Perhaps it is relevant here to point out that Consultant Herbalists carefully choose herbs which are marketed to them as 'tinctures' (extracts of the herbs with alcohol) or as 'liquid extracts' (non-alcoholic extracts). Understanding the diagnosis of the complaint the choice of 'combination' rests with the Consultant and, opinions may differ, but the ultimate result of therapy is cure.

Condition: DYSPEPSIA

❧ ❧ ❧

DEFINITION

Covering the terms *INDIGESTION, ACIDITY, BILIOUSNESS* and *UPSET STOMACH. Dyspepsia* can be described as disturbance of digestion, so common that we have all had it.

SIGNS AND SYMPTOMS

With the more *acute* form of dyspepsia there is usually stomach discomfort rather than pain, a feeling of local tenderness, and there is usually nausea and vomiting. There may be slight fever with headache, and there is no appetite.

The *chronic* form gives a feeling of fullness, drowsiness and discomfort after food. There is lack of appetite, nausea, and sometimes small vomits of mucus and fluid *in the morning,* improving as the day proceeds. The tongue is furred, there is headache and a feeling of fatigue.

A *nervous dyspepsia* or *chronic indigestion* is extremely common, affecting all ages and both sexes. It can be described as a heavy sensation in the abdomen, discomfort both after meals and unrelated to food. There is nausea 'tummy rumblings', heartburn, and a rising of a bitter fluid into the throat which we call waterbrash. There is discomfort from flatulence. These symptoms are accompanied by headaches, fatigue, lack of concentration, palpitation and insomnia.

CAUSES

The causes of an *acute dyspepsia* are, too much food, too rich food, too much alcohol, and poisons, either as food-poisoning of accompanying fevers.

The predisposing causes of *chronic dyspepsia* are, continuing and liberal use of alcohol; smoking; hurried meals and bolted food; excessive tea or coffee drinking; carbohydrates, including bread, cakes, jam, pastries. Infections in the area of the 'throat'.

It is anxiety, worry, disappointment or overwork, which upset the nervous mechanism of digestion, causing spasm or stomach cramp. Flatulence accompanies this process, in the 'nervous dyspepsia'.

TREATMENT

To stabilise the working of the digestion and using herbal therapy, it is suggested that treatment is taken:– (i) *BEFORE MEALS;* (ii) *BETWEEN MEALS;* (iii) *AFTER MEALS.*

BEFORE MEALS

Try taking a tisane or tea of dried *Centaury.* Take 1oz of *Centaury,* pour on 1 pint of boiling water preferably in a teapot. Allow to brew for about 10 minutes, and take a wineglassful, i.e. 4 fluid ounces *one half hour before* meals. If it is too bitter for your taste add a pinch of *Mint* or *Angelica* to the brew in the teapot. This tisane has proved to be good if there is a loss of appetite also.

BETWEEN MEALS

To neutralise stomach acids which can so often lead to ulcers, try to drink ½ glass of milk every hour except at meal times.

AFTER MEALS

A 'first aid' treatment for digestive troubles is a tisane or tea of *Fenugreek* and *Peppermint*. Take 2-3 teaspoonsful of the mixture, pour on a pint of boiling water, leave to draw, and drink as much as one feels is required. *'Settling'* tisanes can similarly be made up with *Chamomile Flowers* using 6 flower heads to the pint of water, *Comfrey* when fresh leaves are available, and *Fennel* or *Dill*, both or either will relieve indigestion and hiccups. Other popular tisanes are *Herb Bennet tisane* and *Mint tea*, as prepared by the Romanies has proved invaluable for nausea, flatulence and vomiting. It is made by using about ½ dozen sprigs of fresh mint or alternatively 1oz of mint leaves into a cup, infusing for about 10 minutes and taking a wineglassful when necessary. Children like it sweetened with honey. *Mint Tea* prepared in the teapot can be served with milk or sugar.

There are many prescriptions for tisanes using the curative properties of several herbs together. Two are listed here.

(i)　Take *Chamomile* ¼oz, *Catmint* ½oz, *Agrimony* ½oz, *Dandelion* ½oz. Simmer all four in 1½ pints of water for ¼ hour and strain. Take ½ teacupful after meals three times a day.

and

(ii)　A popular second tisane is:–

Agrimony ½oz, *Bogbean* ½oz, *Centaury* ½oz, *Raspberry Leaves* ½oz. Taking ½oz of each they are boiled in a quart of water for 10 minutes, strained and as above ½ teacupful is taken about 3 times a day.

A *nervous dyspepsia* responds well to *Centaury* tisane prepared as previously described and taken before meals.

DIET

Certain foods are irritating to the stomach and bowels, and some tend to produce gases during digestion. If you are prone to suffer from dyspepsia try to avoid the following:–

All fried foods, highly seasoned and twice-cooked foods, condiments such as horse-radish, mustard and pepper, meat soups and extracts, sardines, anchovies and kippers, hot buttered toast., rich cakes and those containing dried fruits, cucumber, onions, melon and pineapple, unripe fruit. Chocolate and malted drinks, effervescent drink, alcohol, strong tea or coffee very hot and very cold food. Any food which is known to disagree.

CONSULTANT OPINION

Consultant Herbal opinion should be sought if conditions do not improve after genuine homely or domestic therapy has failed to produce the desired effect. The Consultant would in all probability classify your individual symptoms under the three headings:–

(i)   *Dyspepsia* accompanied by loss of appetite.

(ii)   *Dyspepsia* where flatulence is a prominent feature, or

(iii) *Dyspepsia* of 'nervous' origin.

For a Dyspepsia characterised by loss of appetite, the following herbs are frequently prescribed in the form of liquid extracts or tinctures by the Consultant Herbalist.

(i)   *Irish Moss* (Chondrus crispus) soothing to the lining of the stomach and intestine and nourishing.

(ii)   *Holy Thistle* (Cnicus benedictus) stimulates the appetite, kills germs, and will reduce any fever.

(iii) *Gentian* (Gentiana lutea) stimulates the appetite and improves the muscular tone.

(iv)   *Golden Seal* (Hydrastis canadensis) improves the tone of involuntary muscle such as that of the stomach and intestine and prevents the loss of blood by erosion. It is mildly laxative.

(v)   *Quassia* (Picrasma excelsa) is a gastric stimulant, improves the sense of taste and improves the appetite.

Herbs selected for a *Flatulent* Dyspepsia could include:–

(i)   *Cinnamon Bark* (Cinnamonium zeylanicum). Reduces spasm of the digestive tract, 'heightens' the taste of food, relieves thirst, and gives a feeling of coolness.

(ii)   *Cardamom Seeds* (Elettaria cardamomum). Improves the sense of taste, reduces spasm in the digestive cycle and relieves a 'dry mouth'.

(iii) *Fennel* (Foeniculum vulgare) a favourite in treating children, having a most acceptable taste, reliving the spasm of flatulence and reducing inflammation.

(iv)   *Calumba Root* (Jateorhiza palmata) improving the appetite and removing flatulence.

(v)   *Lovage* (Levisticum officiale) aiding the digestion, reducing flatulence, promoting sweating and inhibiting the growth of bacteria.

(vi)   *Balm* (Melissa officinalis) calming nervous excitement, relieving spasm and promoting sweating.

(vii)   *Peppermint* (Mentha piperita) counteracts vomiting, reduces flatulence and promotes sweating.

For the dyspepsia of *nervous* origin a selective choice could be:–

(i)   *Chamomile flowers* (Chamomile nobile) calming nervous excitement and reducing spasms.

(ii)   *Lavender flowers* (Lavendula officinalis) relieves colic and is anti-depressant.

(iii)   *German Chamomile* (Matricaria recutita) removes the flatulence, is anti-inflammatory and good for travel sickness.

(iv)   *Condurango* (Marsdenia conderango) is a gastric sedative and improves the appetite. It is one of the constituent herbs in the treatment of anorexia nervosa.

(v)   *Nutmeg* (Myristica fragrans) stimulates the secretion of gastric juices, inhibits vomiting and reduces flatulence.

Condition: EAR DISORDERS

❀ ❀ ❀

DEFINITION

The *ear* is the organ of hearing. It has 3 main parts which we call external, middle and inner ear. The *external ear* consists of the ear as we see it, or pinna, and a canal separated from the middle ear by a membrane called the ear-drum or tympanum.

The *middle ear* is an irregular cavity which houses a string of 3 tiny bones which vibrate when sound is passed along them from the drum. It also has two openings, one into the back of the nose and throat by a tube called the eustachian tube, and the second opens into an area of tiny bone spaces known as mastoid cells.

The *inner ear* houses the organ of hearing and contains nerve endings for this purpose which convey messages to the brain for interpretation, but it also has a structure we call the semi-circular canals or labyrinth.

DISORDERS

Disorders include:– (i) *earache;* (ii) *boils* or *abscesses;* (iii) *foreign body in the ear;* (iv) *wax in the ear;* (v) *deafness* – catarrhal or caused by wax obstruction; (vi) *dizziness* and (vii) *travel sickness.*

In considering the *EXTERNAL EAR* we can

(A)   Suffer from:–

(i)   Simple inflammation with redness.

(ii)   Boils or Abscesses.

(iii)   Foreign Bodies such as small beads pushed inside by children.

(iv)   Excess wax leading to obstruction.

All of these conditions can give rise to earache or intense pain in the case of boils, or abscesses where swelling is limited on account of the limited space. Hardened wax, impacted on the drum can cause pain, and the complication of a foreign body can lead to perforation of the drum with much pain.

(B)   In the *MIDDLE EAR* the main disorder is *catarrh* usually the aftermath of a simple cold. We call this catarrh, 'glue' since it interferes with the movement of the string of tiny bones, interfering with the transfer of sound and leading to deafness. *Inflammation* in the middle ear can have serious complications if the infection travels to the mastoid cells, giving rise to what is called a 'mastoid' and requiring urgent medical attention.

If there is little or no response to Herbal treatment with deafness caused by catarrh – after a short period of treatment (determined by the individual) reference must be made to the doctor, on account of the serious nature of the spread of infection in this area.

(C)   In the *INNER EAR* an inflammation or infection can lead to an unnatural disturbance of the fluid which normally circulates in the semi-circular canals, and *balance* can be disturbed. We become unsure of our position and disorientated and can suffer from *dizziness* or vertigo, as in *Travel Sickness.*

This can be accompanied by a ringing noise in the ears, although the ringing noise can occur quite independently of dizziness and is due to temporary faulty circulation of blood in the area.

TREATMENT

We would give a general treatment for *earache,* not specific to any area by giving:–

(i)   Local Heat and Warmth to the side of the face. This is very comforting and hot water-bottle can be used for this purpose.

(ii)   Using *drops* from a mixture of an eggcupful of warm olive oil to which has been added 1 drop of *Peppermint* or *Clove Oil*. Drop into the affected ear.

(iii)   Warm olive oil can be used with an equal part of *Marigold Juice* and using drop doses in the ear.

(iv)   It is said to help if gums are massaged with *Cinnamon* or *Oil of Cloves*.

A Boil or Abscess in the ear is a very painful condition and for local comfort put ¹/₂ teaspoonful of *Peppermint* or *Rosemary Oil* in a basin of hot water and sit with the ear over the basin – the head covered by a thick towel, but the nose and mouth need not be in the same area. The patient should consult the doctor if pain becomes too severe.

A Foreign Body in the ear such as bead pushed there by a child, needs skilled hands to remove it and pointed objects should never be used as irreparable harm can be caused if the drum is accidentally perforated. Warm *Olive Oil* dropped into the ear can sometimes cause a small foreign body such as an insect to float to the exit on the oil.

Wax in the ear. Wax in normally present in small amounts in the ear – it is a natural secretion, but if excess wax is produced it can harden and become impacted on the ear-drum. *Olive Oil* and *Peppermint Oil* prepared as for use in boils in the ear (above) can be dropped into the ear for a few nights in succession and 'worked in' by moving the lobe of the ear in a rotating position, and refraining from stuffing the ear with cotton wool. Do this before retiring to bed and sleep on the affected side. The 'dissolved' wax will more than likely run out on the pillow in the night.

Catarrhal Deafness. For treatment reference should be made under the heading of *catarrh*.

In addition warm *Olive Oil* with a few drops of *Onion Juice* mixed with it has been beneficial as drops in the ear.

Dizziness. Reference has already been made to infection in the inner ear.

(i)   A cold tisane of *Valerian* is helpful prepared by using ¹/₂ teaspoonful *Valerian herb* to 1 pint of boiling water and allowed to cool before taking it.

(ii)   *Apple Cider Vinegar* mixed with a teaspoonful of honey in warm water is a great help.

Ringing in the ears can be aleviated by drinking *Sage tea* – 2 pinches of Sage to 1 cup of boiling water and infuse.

or

Infusing *Hawthorn Berries* and preparing a tisane.
or
Likewise infusing leaves of *Buchu* to prepare a tisane.
The fruit *Papaya* is known to relieve *Travel Sickness,* and drinking *peppermint* tea is helpful.

CONSULTANT OPINION
(i)   *Golden Seal* (Hydrastis canadensis) is frequently used in combination with *Myrrh, Cone Flower, Mullein* and *Eucalyptus,* as *drops* for *ear disorders.*
(ii)   *Elder Flowers* (Sambucus nigra) is taken as medicine for the treatment of colds and influenza, a forerunner of *catarrhal deafness.*
(iii)   *Betony* (Stachys betonica) is a well-known sedative used as a medicine for the treatment of *dizziness* or *vertigo.*
(iv)   *Black cohosh* (Cimicifuga racemosa), combined with *Prickly Ash, Golden Seal* and *Ground Ivy* are used for the treatment of *ringing in the ears.*
(v)   *German Chamomile* (Matricaria chamomile) is a favourite for the treatment of *travel sickness.*

Condition: ECZEMA

DEFINITION
Eczema is an inflammation of the skin due to the reaction of something *on* the body, or *inside* the body in an especially sensitive person. It appears to be a disease of our time as so many new substances become available commercially.

DESCRIPTION
It is probably first seen as a scaly and fissured rash with a tendency to sticky fluid discharges, and can occur on any part of the body and at any age. The rash goes through 3 definite stages of development:–
Stage I: There is redness and swelling which can disappear completely.
Stage II: Raised spots appear along with tiny blisters.
Stage III: Broken blisters, and the fluid from inside the blisters forms crusts. This stage is called *Weeping Eczema.*

The areas can become *infected* and the picture is then one of blisters, fissures and pus. On the other hand the rash may remain at the *chronic* stage where the skin surface flakes and may become thickened in places.

CAUSES
Precipitating causes can be either: (a) *External* or (b) *Internal*.

External Precipitating Causes
(i)   Extremes of weather such as too hot or too cold, or excessive sunshine.
(ii)   The subject can be exposed to certain substances such as metals, varnishes, cements, when an extra sensitivity will produce the skin changes.

Internal Precipitating Causes
The following conditions are known to produce rashes in some sensitive individuals:–
Indigestion, Diabetes, Gout; Allergies, and *Emotional States* such as *Overwork* and *Worry.*

SYMPTOMS OF THE RASH
These included itching, throbbing and/or burning sensation in the area involved.

TREATMENT
Try to track down the offending irritant.
Suspect:–
(i)   Any *liquid* applied to the skin for whatever purpose.
(ii)   *Soaps,* soap and water irritate a skin with eczema, so use olive oil to clean the skin.
(iii)   *Disinfectants* such as Dettol or T.C.P.
(iv)   *Detergents* such as washing-up liquids – always wear rubber gloves.
Background help includes:–
(i)   Do not *scratch.*
(ii)   Have adequate *relaxation* and *rest.*
(iii)   Have a *simple* diet.

DIET

Avoid 'hot' foods such as strong spices, garlic, onions, chocolate and wine, which although they are not responsible for the condition, will aggravate it.

Include these items in your diet:– grated carrots; radishes; asparagus; celery; lemon juice and raw or cooked apricots.

HERBAL TREATMENT

Treatment is divided into three main groups:– (i) *Poultices*, (ii) *Compresses*, (iii) *Teas* or Tisanes.

(1) POULTICES

(i)   *Linseed*. Place enough seeds in a small muslin bag to half fill it. Let the bag stand in very hot or simmering water for 5-10 minutes, until the seeds have swollen to completely fill the bag. Wring out and apply whilst still hot. Repeat several times a day.

(ii)   *Hound's Tongue*. Mix 2-4 tablespoonsful crumbled fresh root or pulverised dried root with a little warm water to make a paste. Spread on a linen or gauze cloth and apply to the skin whilst warm. Leave in place at least 1 hour. Repeat several times a day.

(2) COMPRESSES

(i)   *Burdock*. Boil 1 teaspoonful of shredded root in 1 pint water for 1 minute. Let it stand 30 minutes. Make a damp loose compress for 1-2 hours intervals during the day.

(ii)   *Comfrey*. Place 3-4 tablespoonsful fresh or dried root in 1 pint of water. Boil for 5 minutes; let stand for 20 minutes. Moisten a linen cloth in the cooled liquid. Apply a damp loose compress for 1-2 hours several times a day. Moisten the compress again as soon as it begins to dry every 15-20 minutes.

(iii)   *Marigold*. Take 2 tablespoonsful of fresh or dried blossoms mixed with leaves. Boil for 5 minutes in 1 pint of water. Let stand 20 minutes. Make a compress with the liquid as above. Use 2-3 times daily.

(iv)   *Mallow*. Boil 2-3 tablespoonsful of leaves or blossoms in 2 pints of water let stand for 20 minutes. Make a damp compress with the cooled liquid.

(3) TEAS or TISANES

(i)   *Heartsease or Blue Violet tea* is made by infusing 2 teaspoonsful of the herb in 1 pint of boiling water. Allow to draw for 10 minutes. Then take a wineglassful or 4 tablespoonsful doses 3 times a day.

In small children with infantile eczema use *Blue Violet Tea* instead of water to drink. Older children and adults should take the tea for about 4 weeks.

(ii)   *Marigold Tea.* Use 1oz of the flower heads to 1 pint of boiling water, and infuse. Take wineglassful doses 2-3 times a day. This tea could also be used as a *cold wash* for the skin.

OTHER SUGGESTIONS

(i)   *Slippery Elm and Honey.* Mix a dessertspoonful of *Slippery Elm Powder* with the same amount of Honey, and 3 dessertspoonsful of water. Add a pinch of *Cayenne Pepper.* Take this mixture every morning before breakfast.

(ii)   Avoid soaps with animal fats in them. Use *Slippery Elm Soap* or any pure *Herbal Soap* – eczema rashes do not take kindly to ordinary soaps and water and the area may have to be cleaned with olive oil.

CONSULTANT OPINION

Consultant Herbalists may choose to use any of the following Herbal therapies.

(i)   *Mountain Grape* (Berberis aquafolium). It is specially indicated in treating skin eruptions when combined with *Burdock Root* and *Yellow Dock Root.*

(ii)   *Common Fumitory* (Fumaria officinalis). Valuable in the treatment of chronic eczema combined with *Yellow Dock Root* and *Goosegrass.*

(iii)   *Golden Seal* (Hydrastis canadensis). Used as an ointment combined with *Witch Hazel leaf* and *Passion Flower* it has a wide application for a chronic eczema which is complicated with itching.

(iv)   *Common Figwort* (Scrophularia nodosa), also has a valuable place combined with *Yellow Dock Root,* in chronic eczema cases where there is much irritation.

(v)   *Chickweed* (Stellaria media) is contained in ointments for eczema.

(vi)   *Red Clover Flowers* (Trifolium pratense). Combines well with *Yellow Dock* in ointment form for this condition.

(vii) *Stinging Nettle* (Urtica dioica). Specifically indicated in cases of 'nervous' eczema and in the infantile eczema of very young children, it combines well with *Burdock Root* in treating these cases.

(viii) *Blue Violet* (Viola tricolor) is used with very good effect in cases of skin eruptions which are 'weeping'.

Condition: EYE DISORDERS

❀ ❀ ❀

DEFINITION

The *eye* is the organ of vision. It can be described as an automatic camera which registers and interprets its pictures in the brain. Eyes are the most overworked and generally neglected part of the human body and many troubles can assail them.

Dealing with disorders of the eye is in the main the province of the Doctor. The unimaginative do not realise how valuable our sight is until it becomes affected, and the care of the eyes is a difficult proposition. The eye is one of the most delicate organs of the body, and in treating eye disorders it is quite easy to do more harm than good.

Therefore mention will be made of common conditions affecting the eye and its various parts, but treatment will be limited to those conditions which readily clear up with attention.

A.   We have disorders of *the eye itself* giving us eyestrain, inflammation and foreign body, such as grit in the eye, giving pain and soreness. We have a dislike of bright lights where sunshine is very bright, or we work perpetually in dark surroundings, e.g. in mining.

Or we can experience blurred vision, caused again by a foreign body in the eye, by inflammation, by cataract and a poor general condition, diabetes, kidney troubles, and nerve disorders, and excessive tobacco smoking.

B.   The *eye lids* can be inflamed at their margins, caused by infection and very common in children. There can be infection at the base of an eyelash giving rise to a stye, or again swollen eyelids can occur without any obvious causes and may be a pointer to kidney troubles or an allergic reaction, or again we may have been crying or have a cold. Some infectious fevers such as measles often give rise to swollen eyelids. Our eyes can water excessively if we have a cold, have grit in the eye, or suffer from such infections as measles.

Twitching or flickering of the eyelids can come on without any warning. It is usually caused by fatigue and general muscular weakness in the elderly. It is not serious.

C.   Inflammation of the *Covering of the eyeball* is called *Conjunctivitis*. The eye is sore, indeed painful, 'bloodshot' and 'waters' profusely. There is also a dislike of bright lights.

D.   When the *lens of the eye* loses its transparency we call the condition cataract. This disorder is commonest in people over 45 years old. The only transient eye disorders which I consider we can justifiably treat with Herbal Therapy fall under the heading:– *EYE STRAIN: INFLAMMATION: STYES AND CONJUNCTIVITIS.*

TREATMENT

(i)   One Pharmaceutical firm today, prepares an *Eye Lotion* and *Eye Drops* of *distilled Witch Hazel*. These preparations are very popular.

They are reputed to be soothing, cooling, refreshing and gently antiseptic.

Witch Hazel preparations are valuable in the herbal treatment of *eye strain* and all forms of *inflammation*.

(ii)   *Eyebright* (Euphrasia officinalis) is also a very popular choice. The Romanies will use nothing else and they prepare an eyebright lotion by putting a teaspoonful of the dried herb in a teacupful of boiling water, and allowing it to cool before use. They use it for *eye strain*, and when they treat *styes*. They bathe the affected eye lid with the lotion as often as possible.

(iii)   *Ragwort* (Senecio jacobaea) is used in an ointment prepared from the fresh herb and is excellent for *inflammation* of the eyes.

(iv)   The mucilage of *Quince Seed* (Pyrus cydonia) makes a very soothing eye lotion for *eye strain*.

(v)   *Poke Root* (Phytolacca decandra) has proved of much value in treating *Conjunctivitis*.

(vi)   *Chickweed* (Stellaria media) is one of the most valuable herbs for healing *styes*. The freshly-washed herb is placed on the eye and bandaged into place, left for about 3 hours and replaced after 1 hour. *Chickweed Tea* can be made using 1oz of herb to 1 pint of water. *Chickweed Leaves* can be eaten in salads.

(vii)   *Groundsel* (Senecio vulgaris) can be used in the treatment of *inflammation*. The crushed leaves are applied to the closed eye, bandaged in place and left on. In severe cases the groundsel can be mixed with warm milk before applying.

(viii) The inhabitants of Columbria (S. America) have great faith in the use of *lemon juice* as a cure for *inflammation*. A little of the juice is dropped into the eye.

(ix)   *Golden Seal* (Hydrastis canadensis) is used as a treatment in many eye infections and as a general *cleansing agent*.

Herbs used in the past include *Greater Celandine* (Chelidonium majus); *Purple Loosestrife* (Lythrium salicaria); *Fennel* (Foeniculum officinale) which at one time had a reputation for improving sight, and is creeping back into the pharmacopoea; *Pimpernel* (Anagallis arvensis) and *Centaury* (Erythraea centaurium).

A special herbal remedy for *inflammation* of the eye is as follows:–

Take 1oz *Raspberry Leaves*.

   1oz *Marshmallow Herb*.

   ¹/₂oz *Groundsel*.

Put the mixed herbs into 1¹/₂ pints of boiling water. Simmer gently until 1 pint remains. When cold, strain and use as a lotion in an eye bath.

DIET

Include the following items in the diet whenever possible:- honey, yoghurt, black molasses, parsley and watercress.

Increase the vitamin intake especially vitamins A, B and D for *eye strain*.

CONSULTANT OPINION

Other experts in Herbal Medicine would possibly include any of the following herbs in their preparations:–

(i)   *Common Marigold* (Calendula officinalis) used in combination with Witch Hazel.

(ii)   *Eyebright* (Euphrasia officinalis). It is an astringent herb and used as an anti-inflammatory eye lotion for conjunctivitis. It is often used combined with *Witch Hazel* and *Golden Seal*.

(iii)   *Common Fumitory* (Fumaria officinalis) holds a popular place.

(iv)   *Fennel* (Foeniculum officinale). Used as an eye wash in conjunctivitis and inflammation of the eyelids.

(v)   *Golden Seal* (Hydrastis canadensis). Used combined with *Witch Hazel leaf* and *Eyebright* as an eye lotion.

(vi)   *Raspberry leaves* (Rubus idaeus). Often combined with *Eyebright* to enhance the quality.

Condition: FEVER

❀ ❀ ❀

DESCRIPTION

Fever is a condition where the body temperature is raised above that which is normal. Normal Body Temperature is 98.4°F or 36.9°C, and registers the balance between the heat produced in the body by its chemical functions, i.e. metabolism, and the heat normally lost through the skin, in the breath, and in the body excretions. This remains *constant* in health.

Fever is one of the most constant and reliable signs in infections, and is probably caused by the toxic products, i.e. poisons circulating in the body and which are produced by the infecting organisms. The presence of fever shows the human body is giving battle to invading alien organisms, and the effort in fighting them weakens the body.

Fever is graded (i) 100°F – 37.8° Celsius – Slight.

(ii) 102°F – 38.9° Celsius – Moderate.

(iii) 105°F – 40.6° Celsius – Dangerously high.

SYMPTOMS

Symptoms which accompany fever are:–

(i) Chilly sensation; (ii) Shivering; (iii) Feeling boiling hot; (iv) Usually dry; (v) May be sweating; (vi) Headache; (vii) Restlessness; (viii) Furred tongue; (ix) Highly coloured urine; (x) Confusion of thought and speech. Could be delirious; (xi) Convulsions or vomiting in children.

The more *common* causes of fever include:–

Colds, Flu, Sinusitis, Tonsillitis, Laryngitis, Bronchitis, Gastro-Enteritis, Ear Infections and Kidney Infections. We can however classify fevers into 4 types:–

(i)   Fever with a skin rash.

(ii)   Fever without a rash.

(iii)   Fever in which temperatures rise and fall and rise again.

(iv)   Prolonged fevers.

TREATMENT

The principle of treatment is to try to *lessen* the fever a little, but never to *suppress* it. When there is a *feverish* condition and you are not sure what it is, never panic since the presence of a fever means that the body is giving battle. Should the fever persist or alter its character for the worse, then your doctor should be consulted, since fevers falling into the types indicated above may eventually have other complicated manifestations.

First line herbal treatment include:–

(i)   *Lemon and honey.* Make the lemon juice and honey as strong or weak as thought necessary, and take it as often as you like.

(ii)   *Elderberry flowers and Lime flowers.* This combination is excellent to promote sweating, to relieve the body of its poisons. Mix equal quantities of each herb, take 1 heaped teaspoonful, pour on a cup of boiling water. Leave for 10 minutes, then take a cupful 2-3 times per day.

(iii)   *Lime flowers.* These can be used alone to promote sweating using 1 teaspoonful to a cupful of boiling water and infusing for 10 minutes.

(iv)   *Apple Cider Vinegar* and *Honey* is a popular combination for use in fevers.

(v)   *Balm Tea.* Take 2 teaspoonsful of chopped balm leaves, pour on a cupful of boiling water, leave for 10 minutes then take cupsful as required. This tea has the added advantage of 'calming the nerves'.

(vi)   *Yarrow Tea.* Use 1 teaspoonful of the herb to a pint of boiling water and infuse. Take wineglassful doses 3 times per day.

(vii)   *Marigold Flower Tea*

and

(viii) *Tansy Tea* are both popular tisanes.

CONSULTANT OPINION

The most popular herbs used by the Consultant Herbalist to treat fevers are:–

(i)   *Wood Sage* (Teucrium scorodonia). It is used combined with *Yarrow, Peppermint,* and *Elderberry Flowers.*

(ii)   *Lime Flowers* (Tilia platyphyllos). Combined with *Elderberry Flowers,* and dispensed in the form of tinctures, has high popularity.

Condition: FLATULENCE – WIND

DEFINITION
Flatulence is distension by gas which escapes either upwards or downwards.

CAUSES
A. In the *stomach*. This may cause either hiccups or palpitation.
(i) *Air Swallowing*. This is by far the most common cause and can lead to severe belching.
(ii) *Chromic Gastritis*. Inflammation of the stomach lining.
(iii) *Indiscretion of Diet*. Particularly after being on a diet.
(iv) *Gall Bladder Trouble*. Worse after eating fatty foods.
(v) *Hiatus Hernia*. Hernia of the stomach through the diaphragm at the point where the oesophagus joins the stomach.
(vi) *Stomach Ulcer.*
(vii) *Cancer* of the stomach.
(viii) *Faulty emptying of the stomach,* when the process of digestion leads to formation of gas.

B. *In the Gut* (Bowel)
(i) *Air Swallowing*. Gas passes all the way down.
(ii) *Constipation*. Normal gases in the stomach are dammed up by the faecal masses.
(iii) *Excessive use of laxatives*. Undigested food is hurried along too quickly. Decomposition with the production of gas takes place in the large bowel (colon), producing gas.
(iv) *Milk, Sugars, Starches*. Can all ferment in the digestive tract.
'Allergies' or Sensitivity to certain kinds of foods in some individuals cause flatulence in both stomach and gut.

SIGNS AND SYMPTOMS
Flatulence can be so severe as to cause obvious distension of the abdomen, sometimes accompanied by much pain. In young children it is a cause of fretfulness and restlessness.

TREATMENT

(i)   *Herbal Teas* made from *Aniseed, Peppermint, Fennel, Ginger, Caraway, Coriander* and *Sage* are very popular. In this country, these are not mixed together but *separately*, whilst on the continent, the thinking is to combine them with *Coriander, Ginger,* or *Thyme*, only ½oz of the herb is used to be infused with 1 pint of boiling water.

With *Aniseed* and *Fennel* the seeds are used. They are crushed or bruised if possible before being used. *Aniseed* is a gentle and pleasant carminative, i.e. dispelling the gas. It not only helps in the cases of indigestion with gas formation, but tends also to act as a mild laxative.

(ii)   *Apple Cider Vinegar* with or without the addition of honey has proved of great value in dispelling flatulence.

CONSULTANT OPINION

Herbal Consultants might make a choice of the following herbs in their preparations to treat flatulence:–

(i)   *Cayenne* (Capsicum minimum). It is used in the treatment of flatulence when there is no accompanying inflammation. It is a powerful carminative, i.e. dispels flatulence and relieves colic.

(ii)   *Caraway* (Carum carvi). Very useful where the flatulence is causing pain.

(iii)   *Cinnamon* (Cinnamonium cassia). It reduces the spasm and colic in the gut and reduces also any infective element. It is often combined with *Meadowsweet, Chamomile flowers* and *Marshmallow root*.

(iv)   *Peppermint* (Mentha piperita). Used specifically for flatulent digestive pains.

(v)   *Wild Yam* (Colic Root) (Dioscorea villosa). It is often used for a bilious colic with flatulence, combined with *Sweet Flag, Chamomile flowers*, and *Ginger* in hot infusion.

Condition: FLU OR INFLUENZA

DESCRIPTION

Flu is a feverish illness known from antiquity. It is highly infectious and tends to occur in epidemics in winter. It can affect all ages. Complications from flu can be serious.

CAUSE

Flu is caused by a variety of viruses, and the infection is spread by droplets in coughs and sneezes.

SYMPTOMS

(i)   Onset is sudden, and the general constitutional upset is more severe than one would expect with an ordinary cold.

(ii)   Headache, shivering, and 'feeling tired' are common.

(iii)   Coughing, sneezing, running eyes and nose and laryngitis are common symptoms.

(iv)   There can be nausea, vomiting and abdominal pain.

TREATMENT

Keep calm is the first rule, it can be defeated. Try to prevent complications from arising and keep in bed.

(i)   *Honey and Lemon* juice should be taken every hour.

(ii)   *Cinnamon* and hot *Milk* makes a nice drink.

(iii)   *Salt Water Gargles* are excellent. They should be repeated frequently.

(iv)   *Mustard Baths.* 2 teaspoonfuls dried *mustard* powder to a bath, plus a pinch of *cayenne* bring feelings of relief.

(v)   Make liberal use of *Eucalyptus Oil* to inhale. *'Olbas'* is a brand pure plant oils and contains *Cajuput Oil B.P.C., Clove Oil B.P., Eucalyptus Oil B.P.C., Menthol B.P., Peppermint Oil B.P.,* and *Wintergreen Oil B.P.* It is manufactured in Great Britain and is readily available at Health Stores. Use drops of this 'combined oil' on handkerchiefs and pillows.

(vi)   *Garlic,* however badly it smells helps more than many cures.

(vii) The first *Herbal Tea* for flu sufferers should be:–

½oz *Elderberry Flowers*

½oz *Peppermint*

½oz *Yarrow*

Put into a teapot, pour on 1½ pints of boiling water. Leave for 10 minutes. Sweeten only with honey, drink as much as you like.

(viii) An old *herbal* recipe is as follows:–

1oz *Boneset*

1oz *Mullein*

1oz *Sage*

1oz *Vervain*

1oz *Yarrow*

Mix the herbs and put them in 2 quarts boiling water. Simmer gently until only half the quantity, i.e. 1 quart remains. When cool take 1 wineglassful every 3 hours.

All handkerchiefs should be *disinfected* and all *phlegm* coughed up should be *burned*.

CONSULTANT OPINION
Refer to *FEVERS* and *COLDS*.

Condition: GALL-BLADDER DISEASE

DEFINITION
The *gall-bladder* is a little bag in which bile is collected from the liver. The bile is concentrated here, and when the small intestine signals that food has arrived from the stomach, a fixed amount of bile is delivered into the small intestine through a small canal called the bile duct, and bile helps to digest fats in the food.

CONDITIONS AFFECTING THE GALL-BLADDER
There are 4 main conditions:–
(i)   *Gallstones* (Cholelithiasis).
(ii)   *'Attacks' of Gallstones – Biliary Colic.*
(iii) *Chronic Cholecystitis* (Chronic inflammation of the lining of the gall-bladder).
(iv)   *Acute Cholecystitis* (acute inflammation of the lining).

SIGNS AND SYMPTOMS
(i)   *GALLSTONES* (Cholelithiasis).
'Silent gallstones' produce *no* symptoms.
If the bile in the gall-bladder is concentrated too much, *gallstones* are formed there, and are made chiefly of cholesterol. These stones may remain in the gall-bladder and be symptomless.
Should a stone be of such a size to be passed down the bile duct for a distance and then be held up, symptoms do arise. Some small gallstones can find their way out into the small intestine and produce no symptoms whatsoever.

If one becomes aware that the working of the gall-bladder may be periodically 'faulty' one should look to the diet – it probably contains too much fat, or again consider if obesity is present.

(ii) *'ATTACKS' OF GALLSTONES –BILIARY COLIC.*
Biliary Colic is caused by a stone passing 'unwillingly' down the bile duct – it gives rise to agonising pain, with nausea, vomiting, sweating and an inability to keep still.
The *pain* usually starts high up in the abdomen and shoots up towards the right shoulder-blade. The *bile* which is prevented from passing into the small intestine on account of the obstruction of the stone in its path, passes backwards into the body system and produces *jaundice,* a yellow colour of the skin which usually produces irritation or itching.
The *motions* become pale and clay coloured. Blocking the escape of bile may sometimes give rise to inflammation of the lining of the gall-bladder called *cholecystitis* and can be either *chronic* or *acute.*

(iii) *CHRONIC CHOLECYSTITIS* (Chronic inflammation of the lining of the gall-bladder).
The presence of stones can lead to infection and infection can lead to stones, leaving the gall-bladder scarred and unable to function. *Flatulence* and *Distension* are evident after meals, particularly after fatty or fried foods.
There is heartburn, and transient attacks of biliary colic.

(iv) *ACUTE CHOLECYSTITIS* (Acute inflammation of the gall-bladder).
In this condition there are acute spasms of pain in the upper abdomen on the right side accompanied by a sudden onset of fever, vomiting, tenderness, and sometimes jaundice.

TREATMENT
In treating gall-bladder troubles we use herbs known as *Cholagogues* which have the ability to increase the flow of bile.
Since *pain* frequently accompanies gall-bladder disease the very homely application of local heat, i.e. hot water-bottle is much appreciated and helps to relieve the pain.
Firstly – Do *not* use any *purging medicines,* but try the following advice.

(i)   *Lemon Juice* and *Olive Oil* should be taken alternately, one a few minutes after the other. Take 1 teaspoonful of *Olive Oil,* followed by 1 tablespoonful of *Lemon Juice.* The dose should be repeated at frequent intervals.

(ii)   Pour a cupful of water over 1 or 2 teaspoonsful of *chopped Dandelion* leaves. Bring this to the boil for 1 minute, leave to brew for a further 10 minutes, strain, and take a wineglassful morning and evening. Continue this for a few weeks. It is reputed to be a sound preventative treatment.

(iii)   *Milk Thistle.* Is also excellent, particularly when used with dandelion in equal proportions.

(iv)   Drink *Dandelion Coffee* for breakfast, or indeed any time of the day.

(v)   *Broom Tops.* Take 3 or 4 teaspoonsful to 1 pint of boiling water. Simmer for 10 minutes, strain. Take 1 wineglassful or 4 tablespoonsful.

(vi)   *Peppermint, Marigold* and *Horehound,* all made as tisanes. 1oz to 1 pint using fresh herb or 1 teaspoonful to 1 pint using dried herb. These may be used either alone or in mixture.

(vii)   Another *very old and well tried remedy* was to take $\frac{1}{2}$oz of each of the following herbs:– *Parsley Piert, Pellitory, Marshmallow, Wild Carrot, Yarrow, Meadowsweet* and *Gravel Root.* Boil the whole in 1 quart of water for 10 minutes, strain, sweeten with 4ozs Honey, bottle and take a wineglassful 2-3 times a day.

CONSULTANT OPINION

The Herbal Consultant will probably choose a combination of herbs from this list in the preparation of treatment. These herbs are known as *cholagogues,* and are reputed to stimulate the liver to increase the flow of bile, thereby preventing excess concentration of bile in the gall-bladder.

(i)   *Barberry Bark* (Berberis vulgaris). It is often combined with *Fringe-Tree Bark* and *Black Root* (see below).

(ii)   *Balmony* (Chelone glabra). Its use is indicated where there is inflammation and jaundice.

(iii)   *Wahoo Bark* (Euonymus atropurpureus). A popular herb with the Eastern Races, e.g. Chinese. It is specially indicated in constipation with liver and gall-bladder troubles.

(iv)   *Wild Yam* (Dioscorea villosa). So useful in the treatment of biliary colic. Its other name frequently used is *Colic Root.*

(v)   *Dandelion Root* (Taraxacum officinalis). It is specially indicated in inflammation of the gall-bladder with dyspepsia.

(vi)   *Fringe-Tree Bark* (Cheonanthus virginicus). Is reputed to stimulate the liver to produce more bile, and is widely used when jaundice is present.

(vii)   *Black Root* (Veronicastrum virginicum). Valuable in the treatment of gall-bladder inflammation where jaundice and chronic constipation are both present.

Condition: HEADACHES AND MIGRAINE

DEFINITION

A *headache* is a pain in the head and is described as 'the silent cry of the overburdened mind'. It is a symptom of many different conditions and it is not practical to suggest a treatment universally suitable in all cases.

Although a headache is usually considered to be of trivial importance, in a number of cases it can be associated with serious organic disease.

CAUSES

(i)   A *Simple Headache* is usually precipitated by emotional factors, such as anxiety, fear, or resentment. Tension headaches amount to one third of all headaches, and can be initiated by *faulty posture* such as found in the student looking for long intervals at his books, or the *driver*, staring for long intervals at the road.

The pain or headache in the latter cases is caused by muscle tension in the neck and scalp, and is compared with muscle strain in any other part of the body.

(ii)   A *Sick Headache* is called *Migraine* (see below).

(iii)   *Other causes of headaches* include:–

(a)   *Severe infections* such as Influenza.

(b)   *Less severe infections* as in Neuralgia (giving rise to *nerve* pain), and Ear Disease.

(c)   *Toothache*.

(d)   *Digestive Troubles* with flatulence and nausea.

(e)   *Menstrual Disorders*.

(f)   *High or Low Blood Pressure.*
(g)   *Disorders of the eye,* either strain or inflammation.
(h)   *Excessive Eating and Drinking.*
(i)   *Travel Sickness*

(ii)   *MIGRAINE* or SICK HEADACHE

Migraine headaches occur at intervals. They are throbbing in character, and frequently associated with vomiting, and disturbances of vision, such as distorted flashes of light or black spots.

The headache usually affects only one side of the head and is called hemicrania. It may last for many hours and also be accompanied by a feeling of weakness in the legs and a temporary loss of vision. Migraine headaches usually start in childhood and diminish in middle age. They occur more frequently in women, in the intelligent, and in the ambitious. There is also a hereditary link.

POSSIBLE CAUSES

Exact causes of migraine remain a mystery. But *possible causes* include:–
(i)   *Allergies.* Many migraine sufferers find that eating either cheese or chocolate will precipitate an attack.
(ii)   *The Hereditary Factor.*

TREATMENT

Many herbal remedies have a calming and relaxing effect.
(1)   For the *simple, tension* or *nervous headache,* the following treatment is suggested:–
(i)   Rub *Lavender Water* or *Eau de Cologne* on the forehead.
(ii)   *Balm* Tea. Take 2 teaspoonsful of *Balm* (either fresh leaves or dried). Infuse for 10 minutes with 1 pint of boiling water. Drink a sweetened hot cup morning and evening.
(iii) The Romanies have *two* cures,
(a)   *Lady's Slipper Tea.* 1oz herb to 1 pint of boiling water and take a wineglassful when pain is present; also to help sleep at night.
(b)   *Rosemary Tea* with a pinch of *Marjoram* is a good standby. This is called 'lindentee' in Switzerland. Infuse 1oz of herb to 1 pint of boiling water.
(iv)   *Cowslip Tea.* Take 2 teaspoonsful of the blossoms (without the hard base to the flowers, i.e. calyx). Infuse in 1 pint of boiling water.

Stand for 15 minutes. Take 1 cupful.

(v) *Meadowsweet Tea*. 2 teaspoonsful of the herb to 1 pint of boiling water. Stand for 15 minutes and take 1 cupful morning and night. This tisane is particularly valuable for treating headaches associated with *infection and fevers*.

(vi) *Valerian Tea*. Pour 1 cup of cold water over 2 teaspoonsful of shredded *Valerian root*. Stand for 8 hours. Take 1 cup in the evening when needed.

(vii) Ordinary *Indian Tea* with 1 or 2 cloves in the teapot. Drink as ordinary tea.

For headaches precipitated by *Liver Troubles* take 1oz each of *Barberry Bark*, *Centaury* and *Agrimony*. Boil the mixed herbs for 20 minutes in 3 pints of water. Strain and take wineglassful doses 2 or 3 times per day.

(2) For *MIGRAINE*. The following specialised therapy is suggested:–

(i) Rest in a dark room with curtains drawn.

(ii) Prepare a *head compress* of the following:–

5 *Chamomile Flowers*, plus a handful of *Lavender* and a handful of *Balm* in 2 pints of cold water.

(iii) Relaxing and Calming effects are produced by teas made separately with these herbs – *Feverfew, Rosemary, Betony* and *Ground Ivy*, in each case using 1 teaspoonful of the dried herb to 1 pint of boiling water.

(iv) 3 small leaves of *Feverfew* chopped up in a sandwich and taken daily, over a period of months has been known to considerably lengthen the period of time between attacks of migraine.

(v) Infuse a pinch of *Vervain*, a pinch of *Cinnamon*, a pinch of *Basil* and a pinch of *Thyme* in 1 cup of boiling water. Strain and drink.

(vi) Mix ½oz *Vervain* with ½oz *Skullcap* in 1½ pints of boiling water. Infuse or 'brew' for 15 minutes, strain and take 2 small wineglasses per day.

CONSULTANT OPINION

Once again the Consultant has a very wide variety of herbs to choose from in prescribing treatment.

(1) In dealing with the *Simple* Headache they may use:–

(i) *Betony* (Betonica officinale). Valuable for nervous or tension headaches and neuralgia. The combination with *Skullcap* for this purpose is popular.

(ii)   *Hops* (Humulus lupulus). Useful in headaches associated with indigestion and also nervous tension.

(iii)   *Maté* or *Paraguay Tea* (Ilex paraguariensis). Used to treat headaches associated with fatigue.

(2)   When treating the *Migraine* headache the specific choice should be:–

(i)   *Gelsemium* or *Yellow Jasmine Root* (Gelsemium sempervirens) often used combined with *Valerian* and *Jamaica Dogwood;*

or

(ii)   *Valerian* (Valeriana officinalis). When the choice of combination is *Mistletoe* and *Skullcap;*

or

(iii)   *Rosemary* (Rosmarius officinalis). When the combination will be with *Valerian, Gelsemium* and *Sage.*

Condition: IMPETIGO

DESCRIPTION

Impetigo is a skin rash commonly seen in children. It affects exposed parts of the body such as the face, the scalp and the hands. It appears as small red spots which rapidly develop into blisters which break and 'weep' and dry to form honey-coloured crusts.

It is highly infectious. It spreads not only from one person to another by contact, but other parts of the body can become infected by rubbing or scratching.

CAUSE

Unhygenic conditions; Poor general health of the individual.

TREATMENT

(i)   Hygienic conditions at all times. Cleanliness.

(ii)   Nourishing diet.

Treatment of the rash consists of removing the crusts in one of the following ways:–

(i)   Bathing in *warm water* or *antiseptic lotion* (REFER TO ECZEMA).
(ii)   Warm *Olive Oil* compresses.
(iii) *Slippery Elm* or *Starch* poultices.
A *poultice* is made by mixing the *Slippery Elm* powder or the starch to a paste. It must be thick enough to be retained in a muslin bag which can be applied directly to the skin.

Condition: KIDNEY DISEASE

❀ ❀ ❀

DEFINITION
Kidneys are the organs in the body which excrete urine. They are situated in the posterior abdomen. One on either side of the spine. The essential function of the kidney is to remove waste products from the body formed during metabolism, which is the chemical process normally taking place in living cells.
Since kidney complaints are numerous and can be severe, many are beyond the scope of treatment which any household can provide successfully, therefore early, seek PROFESSIONAL MEDICAL ADVICE.
Kidney disorders include:–
(i)   *Acute or Chronic Infections* named pyelitis or pyelonephritis.
(ii)   *Kidney Stones and Gravel* (a popular term for small stones amounting to sludge).
(iii) *Nephritis.*
(iv)   *Kidney Tumour.*
(v)   *Tuberculosis.*

SIGNS AND SYMPTOMS
The signs and symptoms of kidney disorders can be startling, amounting to:–
Severe pains in the back and thighs with a 'dragging down' sensation; distended abdomen and numbness on the side of the affected kidney; difficulty in passing water which may be milky white due to the presence of albumen, or dark red if blood is present; also headaches, giddiness, vomiting and a steady loss in weight.

TREATMENT

(i)   A decoction of equal parts *Slippery Elm Bark* and *Marshmallow Root*, taking a wineglassful dose 2-3 times a day is very soothing when pain is severe. The bark and the root are boiled together for 15 minutes, strained and cooled before taking a dose.

(ii)   Use *Parsley Piert* 1oz of herb to 1 pint of water to prepare a tisane. It has long been in use in cases of gravel and has proved valuable in seemingly incurable cases.

(iii)   *Burdock* has also stood the test of time and combined with *Dandelion* made a fine old country wine.

A useful *recipe* containing both dandelion and burdock is as follows:–

1oz *Burdock Seed.*
1oz *Dandelion Seed.*
1oz *Marshmallow Root.*
1oz *Tansy.*
1oz *Bearberry.*

Mix with 2 quarts of water, bring to the boil and simmer until the quantity is reduced to 1 quart. Cool, and on the 1st day take a wineglassful, i.e. 4 tablespoonsful every 2 hours, then on succeeding days every 3 hours.

(iv)   An old Romany recipe states:–

Take a handful of *Nettles* and a handful of *Tansy* (fresh herbs). Add 1 quart of water. Boil for 10 minutes, cool, strain and drink a cupful at a time 2-3 times daily.

(v)   A tisane of *St John's Wort* taken in wineglass doses 3 times a day has a place in treatment. Use 1 teaspoonful of the dried herb to 1 pint of boiling water. Infuse, i.e. 'brew' for 10 minutes before taking a dose.

(vi)   Likewise, take an ounce of *Couch Grass roots* and boil in 1½ pints of water for 5 minutes, strain, cool, and take in wineglassful doses 5-6 times a day.

(vii)   To help *Gravel and Small Stones* to pass, the following tea or tisane is suggested:–

Mix equal parts of *Birch leaves, Speedwell, Chicory* and *Couch Grass*. Steep 1 teaspoonful of the mixture in ½ cup of boiling water, strain and take 1-1½ cups a day.

(viii) For other *kidney problems,* take *Rhubarb Root* 1 part; *Restharrow* 1 part; *Sticklewort* 2 parts; and use 1½ teaspoonsful in ½ cup boiling water. Drinking ½ cupful before breakfast and 1 cupful during the rest of the day will help to alleviate the condition.

(ix)   The Romanies say that *Broom Flowers* and *Bramble Tops* will cure all kinds of kidney complaints. Take 1 tablespoonful of *Broom Tops,* 1 tablespoonful of *Bramble Leaves.* Brew these with ³/₄ pint of boiling water, cool, and take 1 tablespoonful dose both morning and night.

CONSULTANT OPINION
Consultant Herbalists favour:–
Corn Silk (Zea Mays), and they may use it in combination with *Parsley Piert* (Aphanes arvensis) and *Gravel Root,* or *Joe-Pye Weed* (Eupatorium purpureum) in the treatment of kidney gravel.

Condition: LARYNGITIS

❀ ❀ ❀

DESCRIPTION
Laryngitis is an inflammation of the 'voice box' in the throat, producing huskiness or even a temporary loss of voice. There are 2 types of laryngitis called:–
(i) *Chronic* and (ii) *Acute.*

(i) *Chronic laryngitis* can last for several weeks and is prevalent amongst schoolteachers and football fans and is due to overuse of the normal voice.
Chronic laryngitis sometimes follows catarrhal inflammation of the back of the throat and sinuses, and tonsillitis. Irritating vapours and fumes can sometimes produce the condition, likewise smoking and alcoholism.

SYMPTOMS
The main symptoms include a husky voice and pain in the throat on swallowing; but the individual does not feel particularly ill.

(ii)   *Acute laryngitis* has a sudden, severe onset with fever. The individual feels ill. There is pain on swallowing and difficulty in breathing. Much sputum can be coughed up.
If hoarseness or total loss of voice persists for more than 2 weeks, there

should be professional medical investigation in case the condition is the onset of the more serious conditions including tuberculosis and malignant growth.

TREATMENT
Treatment can be by (a) *gargles* and (b) *tisanes* (teas).
(i)   *Sage* gargle is very helpful.
Take 1oz of dried *Sage* and to it add a tablespoonful of honey and a pint of hot (not boiling) water. Cover till cold, strain and gargle. If a more stimulating gargle is required then add equal parts of vinegar and water to the above.
(ii)   Gargle with *Apple Cider Vinegar.*
(iii)   For the congestion of the vocal cords associated with chronic laryngitis a tisane of *White Horehound* is advised. Pour 1 pint of boiling water on 1 teaspoonful of the dried herb. Allow it to infuse for 10 minutes, then take a wineglassful three times a day.
(iv)   *Blackcurrant Tea* using 1oz of the fruit and leaves to a pint of boiling water, allowing it to brew, then straining and when cool taking wineglassful doses is very helpful.
(v)   *Yarrow Tea* use 1oz of the flowers to 1 pint of boiling water and take wineglassful doses.
(v)   Make a paste of *Slippery Elm* powder using 3 teaspoonsful, 1 teaspoonful of *Cayenne,* 4 or 5 teaspoonsful of milk and honey as required.
Have this twice a day – before breakfast and before retiring to bed.
(vi)   Infuse a *pinch* of each of the following herbs in a cup of boiling water – *Thyme, Mint* and *Mallow,* and take a cupful of the tisane three times a day.

CONSULTANT OPINION
Refer to combination of herbs used in the herbal treatment of Tonsillitis, which have great value.
(i)   A very popular syrup used by The Consultant, specifically for laryngitis with total voice loss is combination of *Balm of Gilead* (Populus gileadensis) and *Pine* (Pinus strobus). It is used widely in the treatment of children.
(ii)   *Red Sage* (Salvia officinalis) is used as a gargle combined with *Balm of Gilead* and *Tormentil.*

Condition: LIVER DISORDERS

DEFINITION

The liver is a large organ in the upper right half of the abdomen. It is the only organ in the body which can regenerate its own tissue. It performs many important functions which include:–

(i)   Manufacture of *bile*.

(ii)   Preparing *proteins, fats* and *carbohydrates* either for immediate use or storage by the body.

(iii)   Along with the pancreas it keeps the sugar in the blood at a certain level.

(iv)   It prepares the substance which makes the blood clot, so that we do not bleed to death if we cut a finger.

(v)   It removes poisons from the body and destroys bacteria and viruses entering the body in the food we eat.

(vi)   It deals with unwanted blood pigment and worn out cells.

AILMENTS OF THE LIVER

(1) JAUNDICE – 'YELLOW JAUNDICE'

When one is suffering from 'jaundice', the skin and the whites of the eye become yellow. We can always look here as a pointer to liver trouble or a disorder of the blood.

Cause:– A blocked bile duct.

SIGNS AND SYMPTOMS

The urine becomes dark, the motions pale, the skin itches, and pain is felt in the upper right part of the abdomen.

(2) INFECTIVE HEPATITIS – 'CHILL ON THE LIVER'

Cause:– Inflammation by a virus.

SIGNS AND SYMPTOMS

The onset is usually slow. There is fever, a distaste for food, diarrhoea and vomiting for several days, followed by jaundice.

(3) CIRRHOSIS OF THE LIVER

Cause:– Failure of the liver cells to renew themselves as they wear out.

The areas involved are replaced by scarring, and this interferes with the circulation of the blood in the liver.

SIGNS AND SYMPTOMS
Dyspepsia and excess fatigue. There is muscular weakness, jaundice, piles and sometimes yellow nodules around the eye.
Cause:– The aftermath of liver infections, or damage from gallstones or chronic alcoholism.

TREATMENT
Diet is very important under this heading and herbal treatment follows along the same lines as that for *GALL-BLADDER*. Refer.

DIET
Salads and fruit should form a large part of the diet. Boiled or steamed fish, lamb or mutton with little fat; lean meat and poultry can all be taken.

Moderation with potatoes and vegetables is the watchword. Wholemeal bread should be eaten. Ripe fruit is a must, but cut down on the intake of oranges as these can cause biliousness. A small amount of jam or jelly is advised.

It is advisable to *avoid* wines and any form of alcoholic drink. Soups and stews should not be taken with full meals.

Tea is not helpful as a drink, neither is coffee but *Dandelion Coffee* and *Cider Vinegar* are good replacements.

An occasional *fasting day* with only drinks of water, lemon juice and barley water has a wonderful effect in 'cleansing' the gall-bladder.

Condition: MENSTRUAL DISORDERS

DESCRIPTION
Menstruation is a monthly discharge of the lining of the womb in sexually mature women in the absence of pregnancy. In the maturing woman, menstruation during the first year of onset may not be regular either in occurrence or duration.

This is normal and does not require any special attention. The character of menstrual periods may differ in different individuals, and periods which are scanty and infrequent, but not entirely absent are normal type.

Discomforts arising during menstruation should be dealt with. They include:–

(A)   *Premenstrual Tension.*

(B)   *Scanty Periods or Total Absence and known as Amenorrhoea.*

(C)   *Period Pains Known as Dysmenorrhoea.*

(D)   *Excessive and Irregular flow called Menorrhagia.*

(E)   Irritability, Depression, Enlarged Breasts, Swollen Abdomen, Headache and Backache, Skin Troubles such as *Acne* which tend to get worse, so do attacks of *Asthma* and *Sinus Trouble.*

(A)   With *Premenstrual Tension* most women feel 'different'. The psychological change occurs approximately one week before the onset of menstruation and is associated with the 'hormone change' in the body at this time.

SIGNS AND SYMPTOMS
There is a feeling of anxiety, irritability and sometimes aggressiveness. There is also physical and mental tiredness.

TREATMENT ‾
General measures include:–

(i)   Drinking less and cutting out salt from the diet for 7-10 days before the expected date of onset of the period.

(ii)   Do not allow yourself to become constipated. Take a mild laxative at this time.

(iii)   Herbs which increase the flow of urine should be taken such as *Rose Hip Tea* (if possible without the sweetening which is usually honey) and *Dandelion Coffee.* Both can be bought at a good Health Store.

Tisanes or Herb Teas have a definite place in combatting premenstrual tension or P.M.T. as we call it:–

Alpine Ragwort; Lady's Mantle; and *St. John's Wort* are valuable in treating general menstrual disorders:–

(i)   Place 1-2 teaspoonsful of *Alpine Ragwort* in a cup of cold water. Bring this to a simmer, remove from the heat and let it stand for 15-20 minutes. Take 1 cupful 2 or 3 times a day.

(ii)   Using *Lady's Mantle* place 1-2 teaspoonsful in a cup of cold water, boil for 1 minute. Let is stand for 1-15 minutes. Take 1 cupful morning and evening.

(iii)   *St. John's Wort* tea is made by placing 2 teaspoonsful of the herb in a cup of cold water, brought to a simmer, allowed to stand for 15 minutes and 1 cupful should be taken over a long period of time.

(B)   *Amenorrhoea* (absent or scanty menstrual periods). In this condition either menstruation has never been established or the 'periods' are in some way suppressed.

There is a period of amenorrhoea in pregnancy for 9 months, and amenorrhoea can occur in other body disorders such as anaemia or glandular malfunction.

Any temporary amenorrhoea other than the normal one of pregnancy in a sexually mature woman should be investigated by a physician.

(C)   *'Period' Pains or Dysmenorrhoea*

SIGNS AND SYMPTOMS

The pain usually comes on about 24 hours before the flow starts and lasts for another 24 hours after the flow has started. It is felt just below the navel and sometimes down the front of the legs, and comes on in spasms. The individual may feel sick, perspire and looks pale. Pain is felt when large clots pass.

TREATMENT

Taking *Yarrow Tea* and having a *Yarrow Bath* are both helpful in painful menstruation.

(i)   *Yarrow Tea.* Pour a cup of boiling water over 1-2 teaspoonsful of *Yarrow herb* or *blossoms.* Let it stand covered for 10 minutes, then take 1 cupful twice a day.

(ii)   *Yarrow Baths* can be either 'sits', i.e. *hip baths,* or *full baths.*

(iii)   For a *hip bath* pour 1 pint of boiling water over a handful of *Yarrow Blossoms*, let it stand for 20-30 minutes, strain and add the liquid to the bath.

(iv)   *Fennel Tea* is very pleasant to taste – infuse ½oz to 1 pint water. Sweeten with honey.

(v)   *Chamomile Tea* using 1oz of *Chamomile Flowers* to 1 pint of water acts as a sedative to relieve the pain.

(vi)   If *Safflower Seeds* are used to make a tea then ¼oz of the seeds are infused with 1 pint of boiling water.

(vii)   *Rose Hip Tea* has a place in the suggestions. Place 2 teaspoonsful of *Rose Hip Syrup* in a cup of boiling water, stir and add a slice of lemon. Drink this for a few days during the menstrual period.

(viii)   Another *Herbal Tea* is made by using:–

$\frac{1}{2}$oz *Pennyroyal* and $\frac{1}{2}$oz *Tansy* to 1 pint of boiling water. Infuse for 10 minutes, then take wineglassful doses 2-3 times a day.

(ix)   A useful *Herbal Drink* uses 5 herbs.

Take 1oz each of *Catmint, Germander Speedwell, Pennyroyal, Southernwood* and *Tansy*. Mix the herbs and put them into 3 pints of boiling water. Simmer for 10-15 minutes, cool, then take a wineglassful, i.e. 4 tablespoonsful every 3 hours.

(D)   *A profuse excessive menstrual flow* is called *Menorrhagia*.

If the menstrual flow is excessive or abnormal even though the 'period' is *normal* in its timing, then we should consider possible causes to be (i) *inflammation* in the genital tract or (ii) *emotional upsets*.

Excessive flow with *irregularity* in the period is considered to be due to a delay in normal adjustment in the hormones in the body producing menstruation and is often associated with a general rundown condition of the body.

SIGNS AND SYMPTOMS

Symptoms include general weakness and agitation; irritability; headache; singing in the ears and palpitation after exertion. For several days before the flow starts, there is a feeling of weight in the limbs and lower abdomen, heat in the passage and painful breasts.

Symptoms subside with the flow, although the individual remains for a while, pale, irritable and run down. Medicinal herbs have a limited, but valuable use in the treatment of menorrhagia. The physician employs far more effective treatment.

TREATMENT

Some relief may be obtained by taking various tisanes:–

(i)   *Shepherd's Purse Tea.* Use 2 teaspoonsful *dried* herb or 3-4 teaspoonsful of *fresh* herb in 1 cup of cold water. Bring to the boil, boil for 1 minute. Stand for 15 minutes. Take 1 cupful 2-4 times per day.

(ii)   *White Deadnettle Tea* is made by pouring 1 cup boiling water over 2 teaspoonsful of the blossoms or the herb. Allow to stand for 10 minutes, then take 1 cupful twice daily.

(iii)   A combined tisane of both *Yarrow* and *Deadnettle* is made by taking 1 teaspoonful each of the herb or blossom, pouring 1 cup of boiling water over this, standing for 10 minutes, take 1 cup twice daily regularly over a period of 3-4 weeks.

(iv)   During a 'bad' session a *Silverweed Tea* will help. Using 1oz of dried herb to 1 pint of boiling water and taking a wineglassful when it is lukewarm and whenever it is required.

(v)   Some prefer *Raspberry Leaf Tea* using the same proportions as for *Silverweed* above.

(vi)   For *Mugwort Tea*. Take 1oz dried leaves to 1 pint boiling water, sweeten with honey and drink ½-1 cupful when it is cool enough to enjoy.

(vii) A *very powerful herbal* recipe is to take:–

1oz each of *Bistort; Cranesbill; Cudweed; Raspberry Leaves* and *Tormentil*. Mix the herbs together.

Add them to 2 quarts (4 pints) boiling water and simmer until 3 pints remain. Cool and take a wineglassful 2 to 3 times per day. Lastly, but not least, a *Tonic Tisane* which provides new energy:–

Lady's Mantle 3 parts.

Silverweed 2 parts.

Woodruff 2 parts.

Tormentil 2 parts.

Cinnamon 1 part.

Mix and take 3 tablespoonsful, bring to the boil in 2 pints of water, let it boil for 5 minutes, strain, and drink 1 cupful every ½ hour.

DIET

Attend to the diet which needs to be rich in proteins, i.e. body-building food, such as meat, fish, eggs, cheese. To combat anaemia through excess blood loss, take *iron* in the form of Ferrous Gluconate. Have plenty of sleep to overcome fatigue, but also have fresh air and exercise.

CONSULTANT OPINION

Although many varying herbs are used by Consultant Herbalists for the treatment of *menstrual disorders*, the following are popular:–

(i)   *Mugwort* (Artemesia vulgaris), often combined with *Helonias Root*, *Pennyroyal* and *Southernwood*.

(ii)   *Cottonwood Bark* (Gossypium herbaceum). Combined with *Motherwort* and *Helonias Root* for irregular and scanty menstrual periods or with *Pasque Flower* and *Black Haw Bark* when there is much pain.

(iii)   *Agnus-Castus* (Vitex agnus castus) a Mediterranean plant which has the reputation of easing pre-menstrual tension, faulty menstrual flow, and painful breasts related to menstruation.

(v)   *Greater Periwinkle* (Vinca major) is specifically used to treat an excessive menstrual flow, and is often used in combination with *Beth Root* for this purpose.

(vi)   *Beth Root* (Trillium erectum) is popular combined with the *Greater Periwinkle* as above, and also *American Cranesbill.*

Condition: THE MENOPAUSE

DESCRIPTION

The *Menopause* is often called the 'change of life' and is a natural process, when the menstrual periods slowly come to an end. The menopause may pass without any noticeable difference, but in some cases discomforts may be experienced.

The 'change' is the beginning of a better life both in general physical health and in mental quietude and self-assurance. The menopause usually starts around the age of 50 years and symptoms and adjustments may spread over a period from 2 to 5 years.

SIGNS AND SYMPTOMS

Over this adjustment period one can experience a variety of signs and symptoms, but rarely does one experience all of them at the same time. They include – hot flushes, redness of the face and neck, hot sweats and cold shivers usually during the night hours. Headaches are described as an 'ever-tightening band around the head' and the pillow always feels 'full of stones'. There are periodic dizzy spells.

Psychological symptoms vary between a feeling of loneliness and depression to grumpiness and fits of general moodiness and bad humour accompanied by outbursts of weepiness without apparent cause.

There may be flatulence and constipation. The menstrual flow becomes irregular, and either heavy or scanty before disappearing altogether. To repeat, these disturbances may vary in intensity or may not be present at all.

One day may be 'stormy', but the next for no discernible reason may be 'bright and sunny'.

The general contour of the body changes, thickening at the waist and giving a middle-age spread. There is no loss of femininity.

TREATMENT

(i)   A favourite Romany recipe for those disturbing 'hot flushes' is to drink *Tansy Tea.*

Infuse 1oz of *Tansy herb* with 1 pint of boiling water, allow to stand for 10 minutes, and strain. Drink as one would an ordinary cup of tea.

(ii)   *Lady's Mantle Tea* is popular. Use 1-2 teaspoonsful of leaves or the whole herb in 1 cup of cold water. Bring to the boil, then let it stand for about 10 minutes. Take 1 cupful morning and night for several weeks.

(iii)   *Motherwort Tea* is made as above and again 1 cupful should be taken morning and night for several weeks.

(iv)   With *St. John's Wort Tea* use 2 teaspoonsful of fresh herb or dried blossoms to 1 cup of cold water. Bring to a simmer. Let it stand for 15 minutes and take one cupful morning and evening for several weeks or even months.

(v)   *Pennyroyal Tea* using 1oz of dried herb to 1 pint of boiling water, infusing and taking a wineglassful, e.g. 4 tablespoonsful doses three times a day as another popular tisane.

(vi)   To relieve all sorts of spasms and lessen sudden pain, make a tea of *Cohosh* (it can be ordered through a supplier), and may go under the Latin name *Caulophyllum thalactroides*. It is used extensively by the North American Indians well versed in herbal therapies.

Use $1/20$oz of the herb to 1 pint of boiling water and infuse for 10 minutes. The dose is a wineglassful or 4 tablespoonsful morning and night.

CONSULTANT OPINION

Three herbs are widely used by Herbal Consultants in their treatment of menopausal 'difficulties'. They are:–

(i)   *Life Root Plant* (Senecio aureus). A North American plant valuable to ease emotional trouble, and hot flushes, and combined with *Black Haw Bark* and *Pasque Flower*.

(ii)   *St. John's Wort* (Hypericum perforatum) is used in treating attendant 'depressed' states.

(iii)   *Oats* (Avena sativa), and included in the treatment of 'depressed' states also, which sometimes accompany the menopause.

Condition: 'NERVOUS' COMPLAINTS OR NEURASTHENIA

❀ ❀ ❀

DESCRIPTION

NEURASTHENIA is a psychological disorder which covers a wide range of 'nervous' symptoms. These include *easy fatigue,* sometimes amounting to *exhaustion,* moderate *depression,* an inability to *concentrate, loss of appetite* and *insomnia or sleeplessness.*

'Nervous' complaints, however, can cover a vast range of illnesses, most of which require *professional* advice. Nevertheless, there are some *first aid measures* which can be practiced:–

They would come under the headings of (I) *Nervous Tension;* (II) *Nervous Breakdown;* (III) *Insomnia* (Sleeplessness); (IV) *Nervous Exhaustion and Night Sweats.;* (V) *Nervous Stomach Upsets;* (VI) *Depression;* (VII) *Heart Palpitations;* (VIII) 'Emergency' treatment for such conditions as *Shock and Hysteria.*

I NERVOUS TENSION

(i)   *Balm* can be considered to be your best friend. Use 3 teaspoonsful of *Balm* to 1 pint of boiling water. Stand for 10 minutes. Cool and sweeten only with honey.

(ii)   A tisane from a mixture of *Basil* and *Sage* is trustworthy. Use 1 teaspoonful of basil to 2 teaspoonsful of *Sage* in pint of boiling water. Infuse for 10 minutes and drink as much as you fancy.

(iii)   *Clover and Marjoram* tisane is very soothing. Take 1 dessertspoonful of fresh *Red Clover Heads* and ¹/₂ teaspoonful dried *Marjoram* to 1 pint boiling water. Infuse for 10 minutes. Drink as much as you like. This is a very pleasant tisane.

(vi)   *Heather and Lavender* tisane is very acceptable also. Use 2-3 sprigs of heather to 1 sprig of *Lavender.* Prepare the tisane with 1 pint of boiling water and use only brown sugar to sweeten.

If the day is marked by a steady *increase in irritability* and *aggravated nerves* try this tea first thing in the morning:–

Valerian 3 parts
Mint 3 parts
Liquorice 2 parts
Chamomile 1 part
Lavender 1 part

Use 2 teaspoonsful of the mixture to 1 cup of boiling water. Stand for a few minutes, and strain. Drink a cupful slowly.

II NERVOUS BREAKDOWN

(i)   *Hawthorn* Tea. *Hawthorn* is a good tranquillizer. Pour 1 cup of boiling water over 2 teaspoonsful of the blossoms or the leaves or equal parts of both. Infuse for 20 minutes. Sweeten to taste with honey. Take 1 cupful 2-3 times daily.

(ii)   Infuse 1 teaspoonful of powdered *Valerian Root* in a cup of *cold* water for 24 hours. Strain, and take a cupful before going to bed. *Valerian* appears to be helpful for most nervous complaints.

III INSOMNIA OR SLEEPLESSNESS

(i)   Combining both *Valerian* and *Balm* in a tisane or tea, make a very good tranquillizer and sedative. Mix equal parts of each herb, take 1 teaspoonful of the mixture and infuse in 1 pint of boiling water for 10 minutes. Take a cupful on retiring.

(ii)   *Hops.* Pour 1 cup boiling water over 1 teaspoonful of *Hops.* Stand for 10-15 minutes, and take a cupful on retiring.

(iii)   *Bergamot* is the 'herb of gladness'. Infuse the leaves or flowers for a sleep-producing drink. Use 1oz of dried herb to 1 pint of boiling water and take a cupful at night.

(iv)   *Passiflora.* Prepared in the same way as *Bergamot* (above) gives a sleep with no feeling of exhaustion on awakening.

(v)   Take a cup of Hot Milk with Honey and flavoured with a pinch of *Cinnamon.*

(vi)   Use a *'Hop'* pillow.

(vii)   A *Mustard* foot-bath is very good to give the body a feeling of warmth and relaxation before retiring.

Use 1 teaspoonful of dried *Mustard* to a foot-bath.

IV NIGHT SWEATS AND NERVOUS EXHAUSTION

To cope with these troubles drink this tisane regularly *after* meals.

(i) *Strawberry leaves* 2 parts
     Walnut leaves 2 parts
     Nettle leaves 2 parts
     Sage leaves 3 parts

Take 1 teaspoonful of the mixed herbs to 1 cup of boiling water. Stand, strain, sweeten and drink. Dose – 1 wineglassful;

or

(ii) *Balm* 1 part
      Hops 1 part
      Valerian 1 part

To 1 pint of boiling water, add 1 teaspoonful of the mixed herbs. Infuse for 10 minutes and take 1 wineglassful twice a day.

(iii) *Dill Seed* 2 parts
       Aniseed 2 parts
       Chamomile 1 part

Use 1 teaspoonful of the mixed herbs to $\frac{1}{2}$ cup of boiling water. Dose – 1 wineglassful;

or

(iv) *Dill Seed* 1 part
      Fennel Seed 1 part
      Peppermint Leaves 1 part

Mix and use 1 teaspoonful to 1 pint of boiling water. Sweeten and take a wineglassful before retiring.

V 'NERVOUS' STOMACH UPSETS

The tranquillizing effect of *Balm* is very useful in the treatment of 'nervous' stomach upsets, because apart from being sedative, balm will relieve cramp and flatulence. *Balm* is good for anyone with a 'nervous disposition'.

(i) *Balm* Tea. Use 2 teaspoonsful to 1 pint of boiling water. Infuse for 10 minutes. Dose – 1 wineglassful.

(ii) Chopped *Sweet Flag Root.* Use 2 teaspoonsful to $\frac{1}{2}$ pint of boiling water and take a wineglassful dose.

Balm and Sweet Flat go together well in a 'combined' tisane.

VI NERVOUS HEADACHES AND SHAKINESS

(Refer to 'Headaches')

Rosemary and *Valerian* are good for Nervous Headaches.
A tisane of *Valerian* 1 part, *St. John's Wort* 1 part, *Lavender* 1 part.
Using 1 teaspoonful of the mixed herbs to 1 pint of boiling water and
infusing for 10 minutes, and taking a wineglassful dose is well advised
for what one would call 'bad nerves or shakiness'.

VII DEPRESSION

Use *St. John's Wort* for Depression. It is a gentle tranquillizer. Take it
as a tisane using 1oz of the herb to 1 pint of boiling water, infuse for 10
minutes and take wineglassful doses 2-3 times per day.

VIII HEART PALPITATIONS

At the first sign of Heart Troubles the individual must go to the doctor
and remain under treatment until healthy. To try to treat oneself for a
heart complaint is senseless and irresponsible.
We do, however, use *tisanes* to calm 'nervous' disorders of the heart or
palpitations.
The following are used:–
(i)   *Hawthorn Tea.* Slow to produce effects and 1 cup should be
taken 2-3 times a day for several weeks. Use 2 teaspoonsful of
blossoms or leaves. Infuse in 1 cup of boiling water for 20 minutes.
(ii)   *Hops Tea.* Use 1 tablespoonful of hops to 1 cup of boiling water.
Infuse for 10-15 minutes. Take 1 cup morning and evening.
(iii) *Lavender Tea.* Use 1 teaspoonful of the blossoms to 1 pint of
boiling water. Stand for 10 minutes. Use 1 cup morning and evening.
(iv)   *Motherwort Tea.* 1 teaspoonful of dried herb to 1 pint of boiling
water. Stand for 10 minutes. Take 1 cup morning and evening.
(v)   *Valerian Tea.* 2 teaspoonsful shredded root to 1 cup of *cold*
water. Stand for 8 hours. Strain. Drink 1 cup twice daily.

IX TO 'CALM NERVES' IN SHOCK AND HYSTERIA

Use *Balm Tea* 1oz of blossoms to 1 pint of boiling water;
or
Chamomile Tea, using chamomile flowers – again 1oz of flowers to 1
pint of boiling water. Infuse in each case for 10 minutes and take
wineglassful doses.

CONSULTANT OPINION

A Consultant might consider *Hops* in the treatment of Neurasthenia or
Ginseng.

(i)   If using *Hops* (Humulus lupulus) a combination with *Valerian* is used as a tranquillizer; whilst
(ii)   In treating a *Nervous Dyspepsia*. The combination would probably be with *Chamomile*.

Condition: PRURITUS OR ITCHING

DESCRIPTION
Pruritus or itching may be either general or local, and instinctively causes scratching.
The itching can either be light and pleasurable, or severe to a degree which interferes with sleep. The sensation 'comes and goes' and is not usually continuous. The skin is often dry and tends to parch.

CAUSES
(A)   *External Causes,* i.e. arising *outside* the body.
These causes we can subdivide into other smaller groups:–
(i)   *Soaps* and other toilet requisites.
(ii)   Certain articles of *clothing* such as *terylene, nylon* or *woollen.*
(iii)   Chemical *dusts* and certain *dyes.*
(iv)   *Bites and Stings.*
(v)   Parasites such as *fleas* and *lice,* or the *'mite'* causing scabies.

(B)   *Internal Causes,* i.e arising *inside* the body.
(i)   *Naturally occurring* itching which passes, e.g in *pregnancy* and the *menopause.* The itching of *old age* does not pass.
(ii)   *Special Sensitivity* to certain *articles* of *food* which can cause itching due to allergy, e.g. shellfish, eggs, milk, pork, onions and strawberries.
(iii)   *Disorders* in *other parts* of the body, e.g. Diabetes, Jaundice, Liver and Kidney Disease, Leukaemias and 'Nervous' itching.
(iv)   *Piles, Diarrhoea* or *Constipation,* and *lack of cleanliness* can cause itching around the back passage. Vulval irritation is common in women.
(v)   Certain skin rashes related to internal body conditions can itch. They include:– Eczemas, and some fever rashes as in Scarlet Fever or Measles.

TREATMENT
Treatment is directed towards searching for the underlying *cause*.
To treat the *symptom* immediately.
(i)   *Almond* – as *Almond Oil* has been used with some degree of success.
(ii)   Bathe the skin with an infusion made from a handful of *Chervil* to a pint of boiling water.

CONSULTANT OPINION
Purifying and astringent agents available to the Consultant Herbalist include:– *Elecampane, Burdock, Mullien, Fumitory, Chervil, Mallow, Dandelion, Hydrastis, Hammamelis, Passiflora, Common Figwort* and *Chickweed.*
A very popular ointment used in practice is *Chickweed* (Stellaria media) combining well with *Marshmallow* and *Slippery Elm Bark* to enhance the local sedative action.

Condition: PSORIASIS

❀ ❀ ❀

DESCRIPTION
Psoriasis is a dry and scaly eruption of the skin. It is a common affliction, and shows as red patches covered by silvery-grey scales.
It can appear as a generalised rash covering practically the whole of the body, but it usually involves the scalp, the back of the elbows and the front of the knees. Sometimes the nails become pitted.
There is little or no disturbance in the general health of the subject, and the rash itself does not itch. The condition is recurrent and improvement may be followed by relapses. These are particularly noticeable during spring and autumn.

CAUSES
Unknown. There is possibly a hereditary link. It usually first appears between the ages of 7 and 15 years, and is very uncommon after middle age.

TREATMENT
REFER TO 'ECZEMA'
Ointments, compresses and teas are used as for ECZEMA.
It is recommended that professional help is sought from a Consultant
Herbalist whose choice of herbs for treatment will consist of the
specialist combinations as outlined briefly under ECZEMA, and
include:– (i) *Mountain Grape* (Berberis aquafolium); (ii) *Burdock Root*
(Arctium lappa); (iii) *Yellow Dock Root* (Rumex crispus) and (iv) *Red
Clover* (Trifolium pratense).
In addition this tea is recommended as a speciality in the treatment of
Psoriasis on account of its *Blood Purifying* and *Sedative* action:–
Take 2 pinches of each of the following dried herbs:– *Chamomile,
Lavender, Sage, Thyme* and *Lime*. Add to the mixture a cup of boiling
water. Infuse for 10 minutes, and take 3 cupsful per day.

Condition: RHEUMATISM

DEFINITION
The term *Rheumatism* covers the variety of disorders marked by
inflammation and *degeneration* in certain tissues of the body including
(a) *joints,* (b) *muscles,* (c) *tendons* and (d) *fibrous tissue.*
(a)   *ARTHRITIS* is the name given to the condition when *joints* are
involved, and here we have two different types (i) *OSTEOARTHRITIS,*
a disorder arising from excessive wear and tear to joint surfaces, and
affecting chiefly weight-bearing joints, e.g. the hip, and usually later in
life and (ii) *RHEUMATOID ARTHRITIS,* where several joints are
involved. There are inflammatory changes in the covering membranes
of the joints in addition to degeneration of the joints involved, and
sometimes this process can lead to 'fused' joints which become
permanently 'locked'.
(b)   When muscle tissues are affected the condition is called
MUSCULAR RHEUMATISM or *MYALGIA.*
(c)   *FIBROSITIS* is the term used to describe inflammation in the
'connecting fibres' in the body and tendons.
(d)   *GOUT or GOUTY ARTHRITIS* is an inherited condition. Here
we have a 'change' or derangement in the chemical processes taking

place in the cells of the body. The result is that excess uric acid is formed in the tissues and gives rise to very painful swellings in the joints, usually the big toe, in an acute attack.

CAUSES
True causes are unknown, but there are several *aggravating* causes. These include:–
(i)   Any condition causing lowered body resistance, e.g. overwork.
(ii)   Nervous or emotional strain will 'trigger' an attack.
(iii)   Long standing colds which have been neglected.
(iv)   Bad teeth and related septic conditions, e.g. gum infection or pyorrhoea.
(v)   Even constipation and poor kidney function have been listed.

SIGNS AND SYMPTOMS
Rheumatism is classed as either (a) *Acute* or (b) *Chromic*.
(a)   In the *Acute* stage of rheumatism there is fever, and pain which is described as 'fleeting' – moving quickly from one joint to another.
(b)   In the *Chronic* stage, the rheumatism becomes localised, there is no fever but there can be excruciating pain, heat, redness and swelling in the area. Movement becomes limited and the condition may eventually progress to deformity.

TREATMENT
Treatment in both (I) *LOCAL* and (II) *GENERAL*.
(I)   *LOCAL TREATMENT* is aimed at reducing pain and swelling.
(II)   *GENERAL TREATMENT* is directed towards ridding the body of uric acid and other body toxins or poisons, and attending to the diet.

(I) LOCAL TREATMENT
(a)   Inflamed joints must be *rested*.
(b)   When the inflammation subsides, *physiotherapy* will encourage a return to natural, unhindered movement.
(c)   *Hot packs* to joints and *hot baths* are advised as aids to both local and total relaxation.
(d)   *Massage the affected areas* with healing oils to soothe the pain and reduce the inflammation. Oils currently used include *Amber Oil, Clove Oil, Eucalyptus Oil, Linseed Oil, Oil of Wintergreen, Mustard Oil,* and these are incorporated in a preparation called '9 Rubbing Oils'

and obtainable from any Health Store.

A well publicised American formula produces another oil for *massaging* – It consists of *1 part each* of *Oil of Cloves, Camphorated Oil* and *Eucalyptus Oil* mixed with 9 parts of *Olive Oil.*

(e)   *Capsicum impregnated wools* are used to good effect as 'packs', e.g. *Thermogene Wool* which can be applied and retained in position for a long period.

(f)   Grind together *Linseed Flour* and *Fenugreek Herb* in a grinder, and with the mixture make a *Linseed Poultice* – quantities depend upon the individual.

(II) GENERAL TREATMENT

Teas or tisanes are used in the 'general' treatment to rid the body of accumulating toxins.

(a)   *Nettle Tea* is a favourite since it is an 'alkaline' herb and 'dissolves' the uric acid. To 1oz of the green tops of nettles, add 1 pint of boiling water. Allow to brew for 10 minutes, then take a wineglassful or 4 tablespoonsful of the tisane 3 times a day.

(b)   *Willow Bark Tea* is very effective. Place 1 teaspoonful of the shredded bark in a cup of water, bring to the boil, and simmer for 2 minutes. Leave for 15 minutes, strain and cool and take a cupful twice a day.

(c)   The Romanies have a well tried remedy for rheumatism. They boil 1oz of *Dandelion Root* in $1\frac{1}{2}$ pints of water for 20 minutes. They strain the liquid and take a wineglassful or 4 tablespoonful doses 3 times a day.

(d)   A teaspoonful of *Celery Seed* in a cup of boiling water and sweetening with honey has a good reputation.

(e)   A firm favourite with *Gout* sufferers is a 'decoction ' or boiled preparation of *Couch Grass Roots.* 1oz of the roots is boiled with $1\frac{1}{2}$ pints of water for 20 minutes, cooled, strained and taken in wineglassful or 4 tablespoonful doses 3 times a day.

(f)   There is a *Rheumatism Balm* which is a traditional herbal recipe and a firm favourite with many:–

For 3 brewings use $\frac{1}{20}$oz of each of the following herbs:– *Yarrow, Wintergreen, Wild Carrot, Figwort, Burdock leaves* and *Angelica.* To this mixture add 1 heaped teaspoonful of *Herbal Composition Powder* (obtainable from any good Herbal Store). Place $\frac{1}{3}$ of the quantity in 1 pint of cold water. Bring to the boil and slowly simmer for 5 minutes.

Strain, and take a wineglassful *hot* 3 or 4 times a day. Doubling the amount induces perspiration which helps to rid the body of its poisons.

DIET
Apples in any form help to cure rheumatism. Drink a glass of *Dry Cider* daily or take a teaspoonful of *Cider Vinegar* before breakfast. The diet should include all sea foods and all vegetables.
Vegetable oils, flour, egg whites, honey, nuts and sunflower seeds. Rice of all kinds, parsley, onions and garlic tea, coffee, and plain soda water. carrot juice and cucumber juice – both can be prepared in a blender help to right Arthritis.
Chicory, eaten as a vegetable is good for gout sufferers.

CONSULTANT OPINION
Consultant Herbalists have a wide use of herbs in their fight against *Rheumatism.* A popular assortment includes:–
(i)   *Celery Seed* (Apium graveolens). It eases pain and has antiseptic properties. It is also valuable in treating *gout.*
(ii)   *Black Cohosh* (Cimicifuga racemosa). In easing pain and inflammation its use is very effective in treating *muscular rheumatism.*
(iii)   *Colic Root* (Dioscorea villosa). Relieves spasm and inflammation, and has a much valued use in the acute stage of *rheumatoid arthritis.*
(iv)   *Wintergreen* (Gaultheria procumbens). Easing pain and reducing inflammation, it has been proved valuable in treating the *fibrositic* types of rheumatism which are *Neuralgia, Sciatica* and also *Myalgia.*
(v)   *Lignum Vitae* (Guaiacum officinale). Promotes sweating, and reduces inflammation. It is valuable in the treatment of *rheumatoid arthritis* and *gout.*
(vi)   *Bogbean* (Menyanthes trifoliate), promotes the passage of urine. It also has the properties of a 'bitter' and encourages appetite. It is of particular value where *rheumatism* is present with generalised weakness.
(vii) *White Poplar* (Populus tremuloides). Is antiseptic, reduces inflammation and pain, and is used in the treatment of *rheumatoid arthritis.*
(viii) *Willow Bark* (Salix alba). In addition to reducing pain and inflammation, it also reduces fever.

(ix)   *Devil's Claw* (Harpogophytum procumbens). Relaxes the patient, promotes the passage of urine, and is valuable in all forms of rheumatism. DIABETICS SHOULD *NOT* USE IT.

Condition: RINGWORM (TINEA)

❀ ❀ ❀

DESCRIPTION
Ringworm is a skin infection caused by a fungus. It appears as circular red patches surrounded by scaly margins.

CAUSES
Ringworm can be caught from other people or animals – especially cats, and particularly Blue Persians.

TREATMENT
(i)   Apply *iodine solution* three times a day – allow the lotion to dry on.
(ii)   *Herb Robert* juice or the juice of *Rue* can be applied directly to the itching patches every 4 hours.
(iii) Apply neat *lemon* juice to the patches every 4 hours.
(iv)   Wash the *lotions* made from any one of the following herbs:– *Yarrow, Burdock, Lavender, Mint, Marigold, Sage* or *Violet*.

CONSULTANT OPINION
Poke Root (Phytolacca decandra). The Consultant Herbalist will prepare an ointment containing *Poke Root* – it is very effective.

Condition: SCABIES

❀ ❀ ❀

DESCRIPTION
Scabies is a skin rash caused by a tiny insect called a 'mite'. The female burrows into the skin where she lays her eggs. The burrows so formed are black, being lined with the excreta of the mite. At the end

of the burrow a small blister or raised lump is sometimes present. The
eggs hatch in the course of several days, and fresh burrows may be
formed.

The commonest sites to find the scabies rash are – between the fingers,
on the front of the wrists and in the genital region, but any area of the
body can be affected.

SYMPTOMS

Irritation is very marked, especially at night when the individual is
warm in bed. Scratching follows, and secondary skin infection follows
with the production of honey coloured crusts of *impetigo*, and these
may obscure the original rash.

TREATMENT

(i)   To get rid of the parasites quickly, take a handful of dried
Buckthorn bark and to it add 2 pints of cold water. Bring to the boil,
boil for ¼ hour, stand for ½ hour, strain, and add this liquid to a
bowlful of equal parts wine vinegar and warm water. Bathe the
affected parts 3 times a day.

(ii)   Soak a handful of *Ivy leaves* in 2 pints of wine vinegar for 24
hours. Strain, and bathe the skin with the liquid.

(iii)   Take *Lobelia* ½oz, *Cayenne* 2 teaspoonsful and add boiling
vinegar, 1 pint. Cool, bottle and bathe the part with the lotion morning
and night.

A *special regime* is recommended for bathing:–

(i)   Initially a hot bath is given and the entire body is scrubbed with
soap and a nail brush. This will open up the burrows.

(ii)   Treatment is applied as suggested.

(iii)   The clothing is not changed for 48 hours.

(iv)   Another bath is then taken and followed by a complete change of
clothing and bed-linen.

Used clothes should not be worn again for 2 weeks and linen is boiled
and laundered.

CONSULTANT OPINION

Herbal Consultants may include the following herbs in their
treatment:–

(i)   *Poke Root* (Phytolacca decandra) is combined in an ointment.

(ii)   *Aniseed* (Pimpinella anisum) is used as *Oil of Aniseed* 1%, and

combined with *Oil of Sassafras* 1% in an ointment base.
(iii)   *Tansy* (Tanacetum vulgare) is combined in a lotion for bathing.

Condition: SHINGLES (HERPES ZOSTER)

DESCRIPTION
Shingles is basically an infection of the nervous system, although it shows as an acute inflammation of the skin. An initial period of severe burning pain is followed by the appearance of bright red areas on the skin which become covered with tiny blisters eventually turning to pus. The eruption circles half-way around the chest, or on one side of the face including the eye. It lasts for about a week but the nerve pain persists for much longer as neuralgia. Shingles is likeliest to appear after the age of 40 years.

CAUSES
The cause is a *virus,* thought to be related to the chicken-pox virus. Precipitating causes include:– lowered general resistance to any infection such as we might find after a debilitating illness, shock, injury of any sort, emotional disturbances, exposure to cold, excessive sunshine and possibly hormone instability.

TREATMENT
Treatment is both (1) *Local* and (2) *General.*
(1)   *Local.*
(i)   To relieve the burning pain rub on *Oil of Peppermint,* or a mixture of *Menthol* and *Camphor;*
or
(ii)   Just keep the area 'dry' by dabbing on *Calamine* lotion.

(2)   *General*
(i)   *Sage Tea* is a must. Use 1 teaspoonful of *Dried Sage* to 1 pint of boiling water. Infuse for 10 minutes, then take 1 wineglassful dose three times a day.
(ii)   *Nettle Tea* – using 1oz *Stinging Nettles,* to 1 pint of boiling water. Infusing for 10 minutes. Then taking wineglassful doses 2 or 3 times a day.

(iii) *Valerian Tea.* Use 2 teaspoonsful of shredded root to 1 cup of *cold* water. Boil for 10 minutes. Leave for 8 hours. Reheat and drink 1 cupful twice a day.

(iv) *Walnut Bark or Leaves Tea.* Use 1oz of the bark or leaves to 1 pint of boiling water. Infuse for 10 minutes and take a wineglassful, equivalent to 4 tablespoonsful 2 or 3 times a day.

(v) *White Willow* can be used either as a *single* herb or in *combination* with others.

(a) *White Willow Tea.* Use 1 teaspoonful of the bark (shredded) to 1 cup of *cold* water. Heat and boil for 2 minutes. Stand for 15 minutes. Take 1 cupful twice a day.

(b) *Combined Tea.* Use:– *White Willow Bark* 2 parts, *Meadowsweet Blossoms* 1 part, *Elderberry Blossoms* 1 part. Take 1 or 2 teaspoonsful to 1 cup of *cold* water. Heat and boil for 1 minute. Stand for 15 minutes. Take 1 cupful twice a day.

(vi) A combined infusion of the following is popular:–

1 *pinch* of each of these herbs:– *Thyme, Rosemary, Lavender, Lime Flowers* and *Chervil* to 1 cup of boiling water. Infuse for 10 minutes. Take 1 cupful each night.

Since *pain* can be very severe and prolonged in Shingles, it is advisable to seek professional help, when the Consultant Herbalist will direct treatment towards restoring general health and improving the nervous debility.

Condition: TONSILLITIS

DESCRIPTION

Tonsillitis or sore throat is a very common complaint which should not be neglected on account of the serious complications which can sometimes occur, such as acute rheumatism and inflammation of the kidneys (nephritis).

It is of the utmost importance that cases of acute tonsillitis should be distinguished from the rare cases of diphtheria, and if there is any doubt about the diagnosis a throat swab should be taken.

SYMPTOMS

Acute tonsillitis is abrupt in its onset. The patient complains of sore throat and pain on swallowing. The temperature is usually very high 40°C (104°F) and is associated with headache, pains in the limbs and feeling ill. The throat is red and swollen and the glands of the neck are tender and enlarged.

TREATMENT

Treatment consists of *gargles* and *tisanes*.

(I)   *Gargles*
(i)   *Sage*. Pour a cupful of boiling water over a heaped teaspoonful of dried *Sage* leaves. Leave for 15 minutes, strain, and use the liquid as a gargle, 3 to 5 times per day.
(ii) *Bilberry*. Add a pint of cold water to 3 dessertspoonsful of dried berries. Boil for 10 minutes, strain, and use the liquid.
(iii) *Tormentil*. Add 1 teaspoonful of dried *Tormentil* to 1 pint of boiling water. Infuse for 10 minutes and when cool use this tisane as a gargle.
(iv) *Elderberry*. Make an infusion of the flowers using 1oz of herb to 1 pint of boiling water. This gargle is very relaxing.
(v)   Save the *vinegar* from a jar of *Pickled Walnuts*. Keep it corked in a clean bottle until it is needed, and use it as a gargle.

II   *Tisanes*
(i)   *Blackcurrant*. Use the leaves and fruit of *Black Currant*. Take 1oz of herb to 1 pint of boiling water. The dose is a teacupful when necessary.
(ii) *Compound Tisane*. Take *1 pinch* of each of the following herbs; *Thyme, Mint* and *Mallow flowers* and add to 1 cupful of boiling water. Infuse for 10 minutes, and take a wineglassful 3 times per day.
(iii) *Selfheal*. Make a tisane with *Selfheal* using 1oz of the herb to a pint of boiling water. Infuse for 10 minutes and take in wineglassful doses 2 or 3 times per day.

CONSULTANT OPINION

A very wide choice of herbs are available, but I will name some popular ones:-
(i)   *Wild Indigo* (Baptisia tinctoria). It is used in a herbal tincture combined with *Cone Flower, Capsicum* and *Myrrh*.

(ii)   *Black Catechu* (Catechu Black) is used combined with *Myrrh* and *Witch Hazel* as a gargle.

(iii)   *Poke Root* (Phytolacca decandra) combines well with *Myrrh* and *Cone Flower* in the treatment of tonsillitis.

(iv)   *Red Sage* (Salvia officinalis) is used combined with *Balm of Gilead* and *Tormentil* as a gargle.

Condition: URTICARIA OR NETTLE RASH OR HIVES

❋ ❋ ❋

DESCRIPTION

Urticaria is an allergic skin reaction which takes the form of localised areas of marked swelling or wheals. They are accompanied by severe itching, and in duration they are usually transitory.

CAUSES

Urticaria commonly results from food poisoning or the indigestion of strawberries, shellfish, eggs, pork, milk or drugs such as penicillin in individuals susceptible to any of these substances.

TREATMENT

(i)   Search for, avoid and *remove the cause.*

(ii)   Local applications to allay the itching, e.g. *Calamine Lotion.*

(iii)   Amusing though it may seem, the best remedy is *Nettle Tea.* Use 4 teaspoonsful of nettles to 1 pint of boiling water and serve with honey. Drink as much as you like.

(iv)   An ointment made by incorporating dried *Plantain leaves* in petroleum jelly (vaseline) is very helpful.

(v)   *Wood Sorrel* is a very effective remedy to use either as a 'wash', or an infusion or decoction, of the herb or root. Use 1oz of the herb to 1 pint of boiling water, and take wineglassful doses. Use the same strength of infusion for the 'wash'.

CONSULTANT OPINION

(i)   *Ma-huang* (Ephedra) is widely used in the Consultant field for allergic symptoms such as urticaria.

(ii)   *Blue flag* (Iris versicolor) is used combined with *Yellow Dock*

Root, Red Clover Flower, Poke Root and *Queen's Delight* with very good effect.

Condition: VARICOSE VEINS

❀ ❀ ❀

DESCRIPTION

Varicose Veins, are enlarged and contorted veins in which valves naturally present inside the veins become incompetent and as a result the normal blood flow is reversed or halted.

Varicose veins are most common in the *lower leg* where gravity tends to 'pool' the blood on account of our upright position. They are also frequently found at the extreme end of the large bowel where they protrude to the outside, and are called *'piles'* or *haemorrhoids*. A cluster of varicose veins in the scrotum is called a *varicocoele*.

The veins themselves may twist and bulge, due to back pressure from an abdominal swelling, such as pregnancy or obesity. The wearing of garters encourages varicose veins and constipation may aggravate the problem. Sometimes, however, this valve incompetence is an inherited factor.

SIGNS AND SYMPTOMS

There may be *no* discomfort felt, but fatigue, aching, itching and a feeling of fullness in the area may be noticed, such as before a menstrual period, or in hot weather, or after a bath or even just after standing. Indeed standing rather than sitting is a long 'neglect' which can precipitate the formation of varicose veins.

The skin over a varicose area in the leg is very delicate and may break down to give rise to a *varicose ulcer.*

TREATMENT

Exercise helps. Do 'cycling' exercises in the bed, before rising, and ankle exercises daily.

(i)   It is sometimes advisable to support the leg veins by means of a crepe bandage or elastic stocking.

(ii)   Where varicose veins appear in the scrotum (varicocoele) the patient should wear a suspensory bandage.

(iii)   For both prominent and varicose veins, bathe the affected parts once or twice a day with *Distilled Witch Hazel* lotion or smear on a *Witch Hazel Gel* twice a day.

Both of these products can be obtained through a good chemist or Health Store.

(iv)   A *Herbal wash* that relieves, consists of:–

Sweet Flag Root

Nettle Leaves

Horse Chestnut Leaves and fruit

Thyme Leaves

Mix together equal parts of these ingredients.

Add 3 tablespoonsful of the mixed ingredients with 1 quart of cold water, bring to the boil, add ½ tablespoonful of salt and use the preparation to bathe the legs.

(v)   As a *tisane*, add:– 1 pinch of *Mint*, 1 pinch of *Sage*, 1 pinch of *Basil* and 1 pinch of *Vervain Lemon Balm* to a large cupful of water. Infuse and drink one cupful each day.

Herbal treatment can be established but medical advice should be sought if any varicose condition begins to deteriorate.

DIET

Essentially a *Fruit and Salad Diet.*

Vitamin E is reputed to safeguard the body against the possibility of having varicose veins, but a dose of 100i.u.'s daily, is a minimum dose to help in the treatment.

Starches and fats (except olive oil) and sugars must be reduced in the meals. alcohol, coffee, onions, spices, sauces, rich foods and tea should be cut out altogether, although 1 cup of weak tea can be allowed at tea-time.

CONSULTANT OPINION

Consultant opinion is directed towards the use of:–

Marigold (Calendula officinalis). *Marigold* combines well with *Distilled Water of Witch Hazel* as a lotion to use locally in the treatment of varicose veins.

Bibliography

Common Plants and Natural Remedies by Cynthia Wickham. Published by Frederick Muller Ltd., London. 1981.

A Guide to Medicinal Plants by Shavenberg and Paris. Published by Lutterworth Press. 1977.

Health Secrets of Plants and Herbs by Maurice Messigue. Published by William Collins Press. 1979.

Medicinal Plants by Prof. Hans Fluck, translated by Rev J. M. Rowson. Published by Foulsham & Co. Ltd., Yeovil Road, Slough, Bucks. 1971.

Living Medicine by Manfried Pahlow, translated from German by Linda Sonntag. Published by Thorsons Publishers Ltd., Wellingborough, Northants. 1980.

Healing Plants. A Modern Herbal edited by William A. R. Thomson, M.D. Published by McMillan. London. 1978.

The Concise Herbal Encyclopaedia by Donald Law. Published by John Bartholomew & Son Ltd., 216 High Street, Bromley BR1 1PW. 1973.

Proven Herbal Remedies by John H. Tobe. Pyramid Books. New York. 1977.

Healing with Herbs by Henrietta A. Diers Rau. Published by Arco Publishing Co. Mc. 219 Park Avenue, South. New York NY10003. 1977.

The Roots of Health by Leon Petulengro. Published by Pan Books, London & Sydney. 1978.

Country Wisdom by Gail Duff. Published by Pan Original, London. 1978.

The Herb Book by John Lust. Published by Benedict Lust Publications, U.S.A. 1974.

Healing Herbs by William A. R. Thomson & Elizabeth Smith. Published by B.B.C. Printed by Belmont Press, Northants. 1978.

Standard Guide to Non-Poisonous Herbal Medicine. Edited by William H. Webb. Printed by 'Visiter' Printing Works, Tulketh St., Southport. 1916.

A Dictionary of Symptoms by Dr. Joan Gomez. Granada Publishing Co. Ltd. Printed in Great Britain by Hazell Watson & Viney Ltd. 1977.